Molecular Pharmacology

Edited by Angel Catala and Usama Ahmad

Published in London, United Kingdom

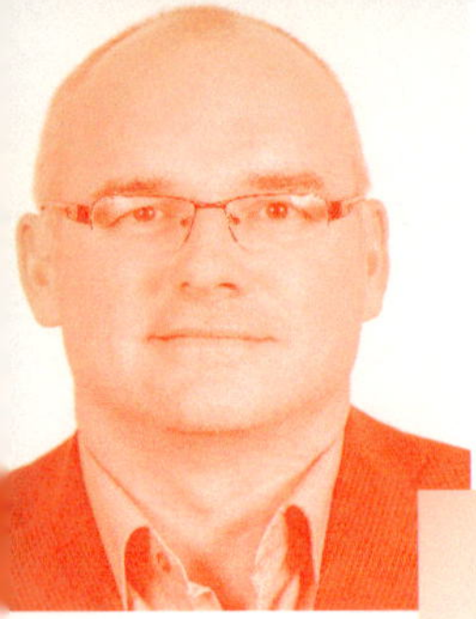
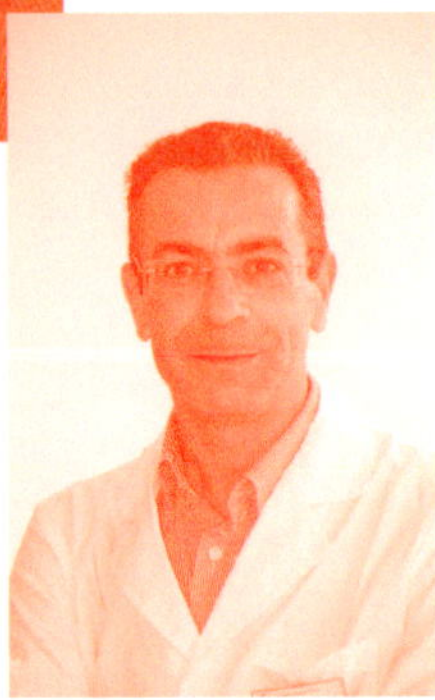
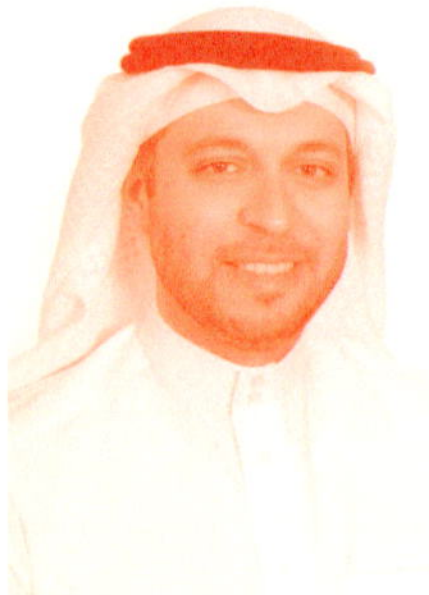
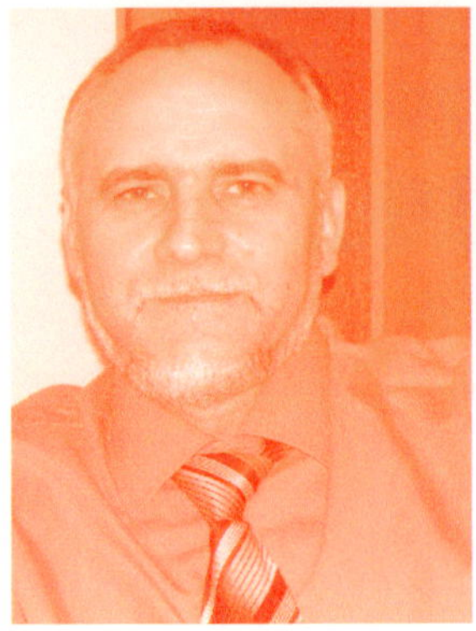
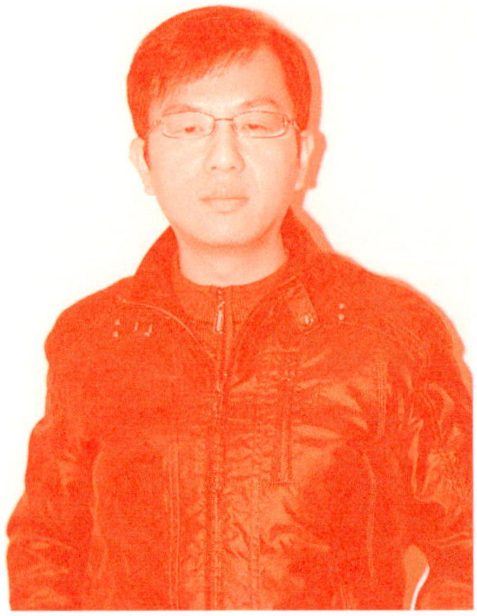
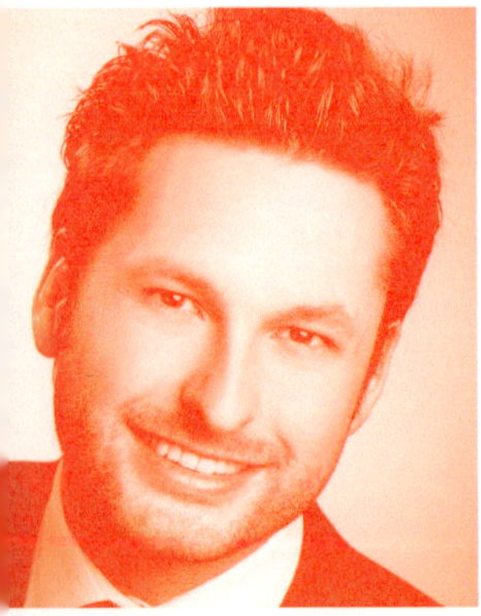
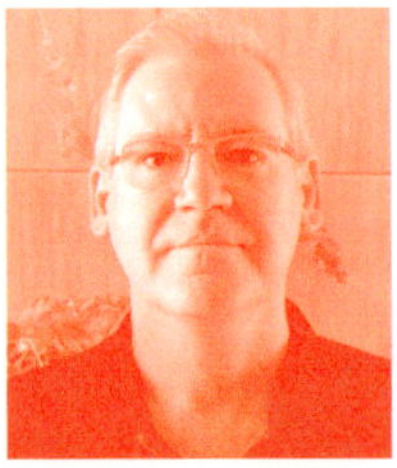

IntechOpen

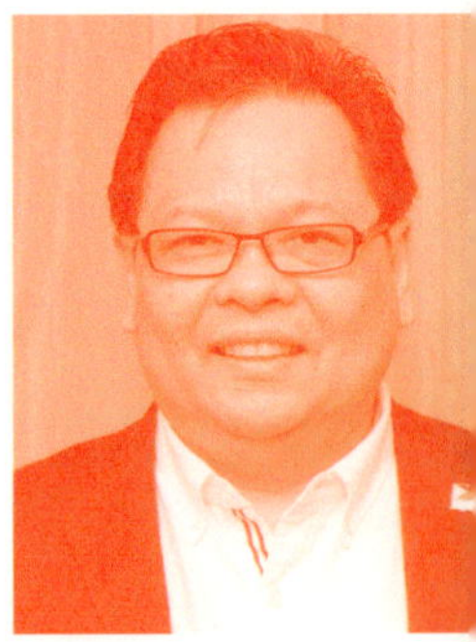
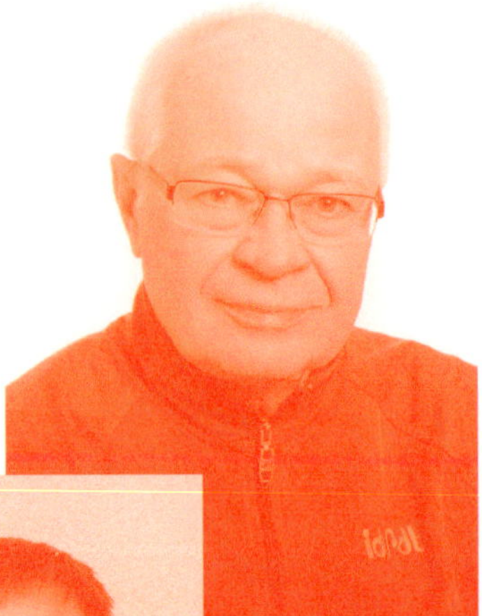
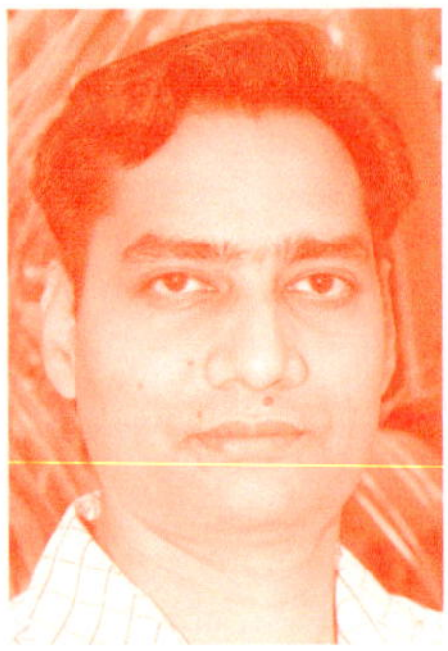
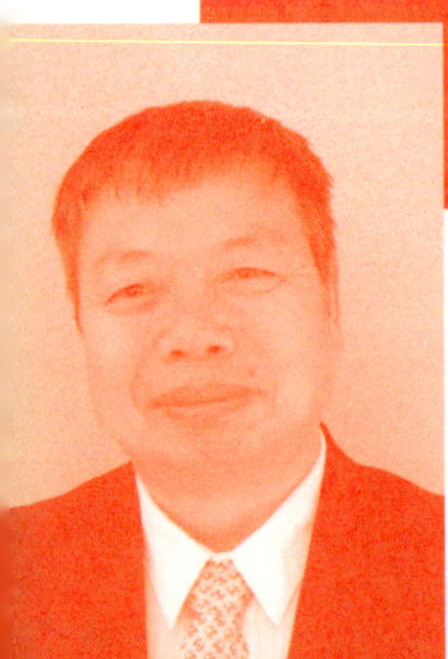
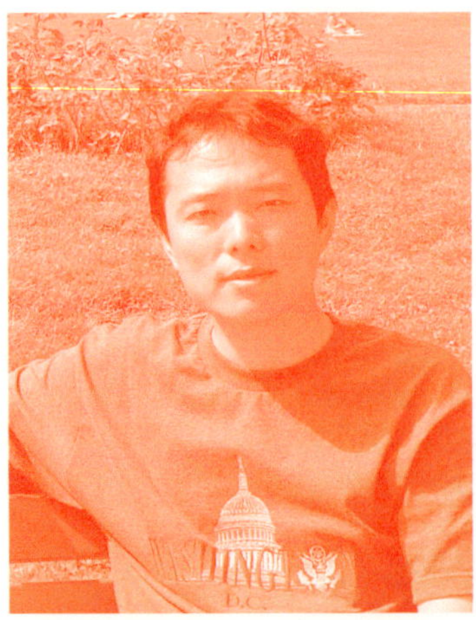
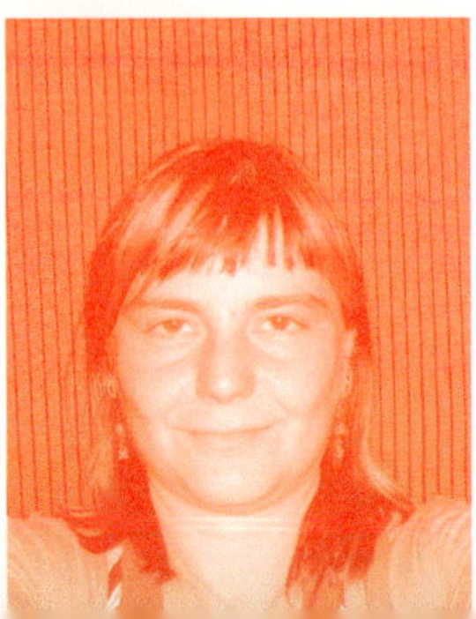

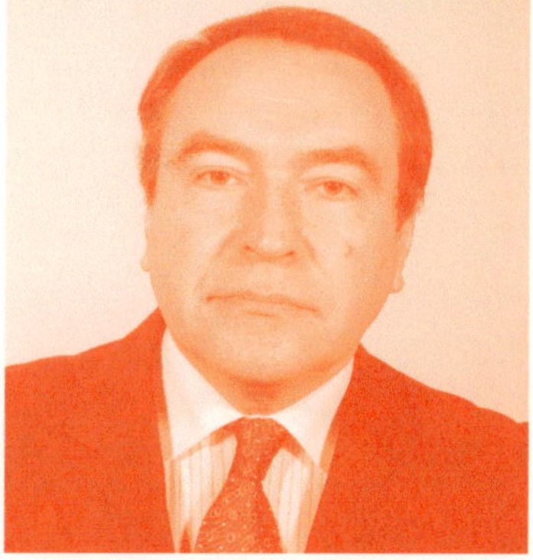
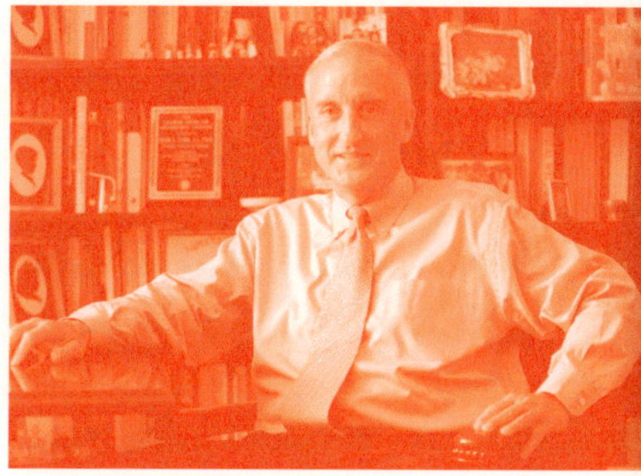
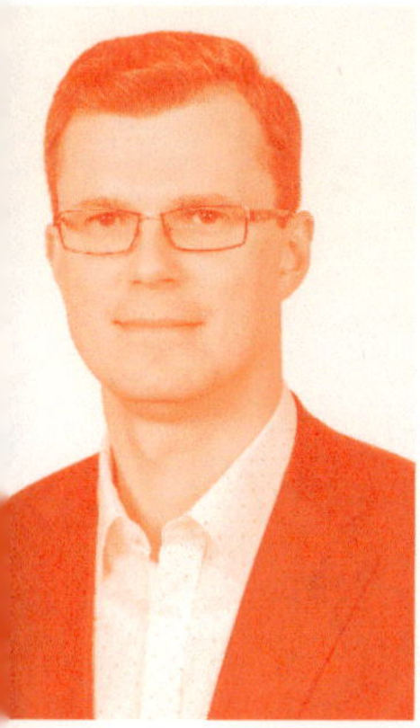
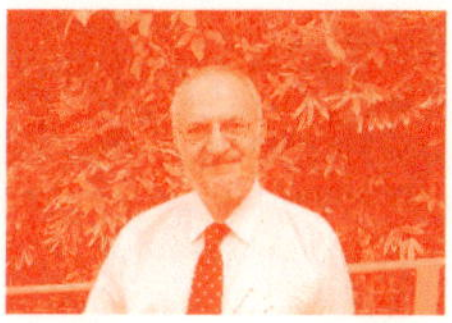
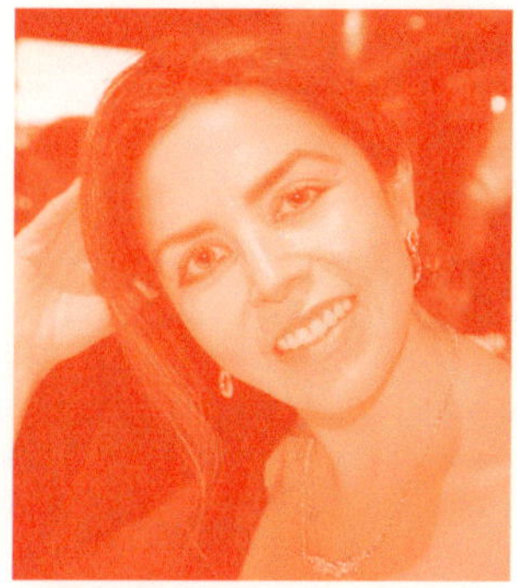

Supporting open minds since 2005

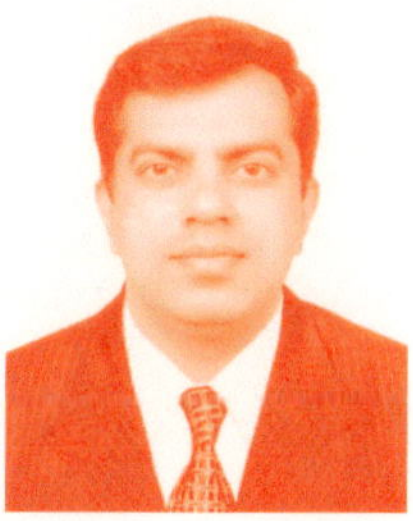
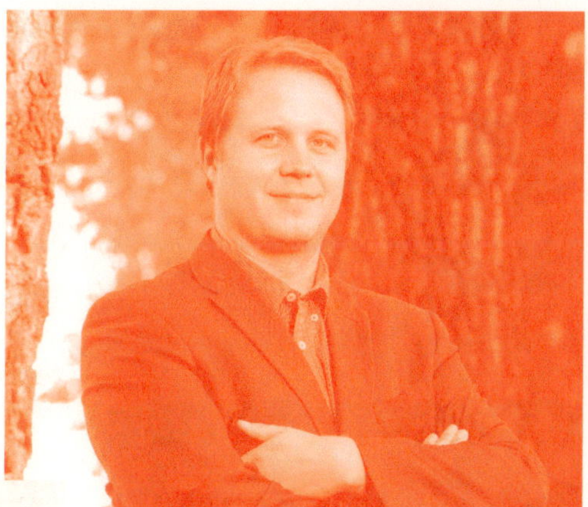
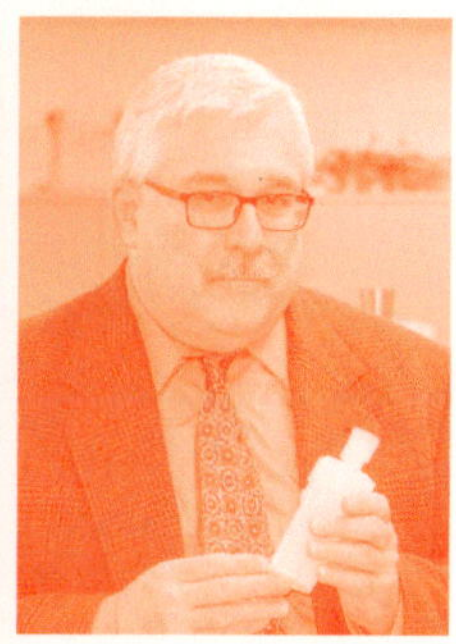
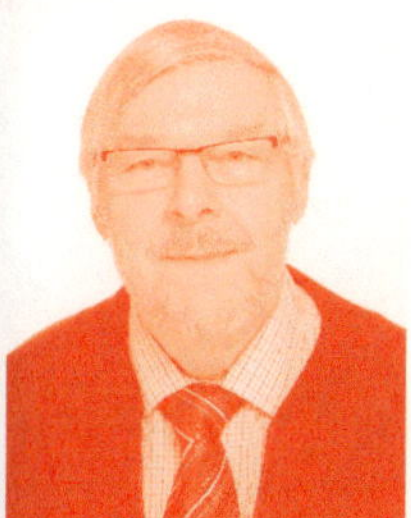
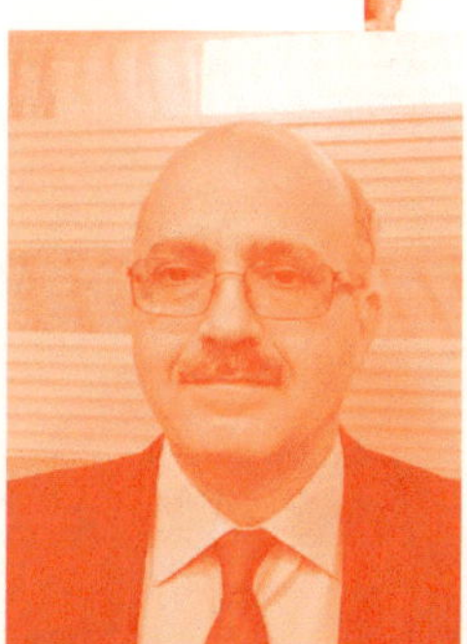
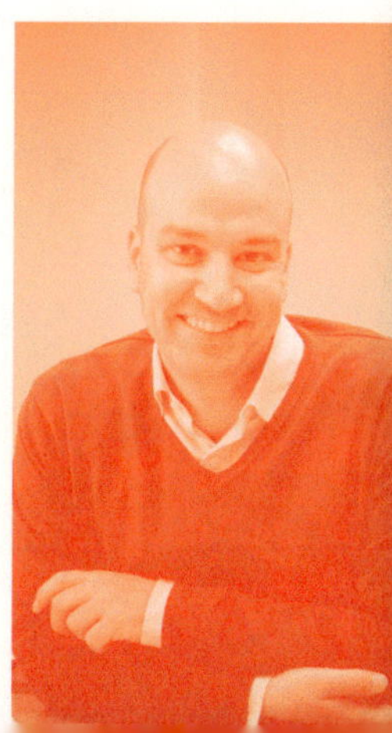
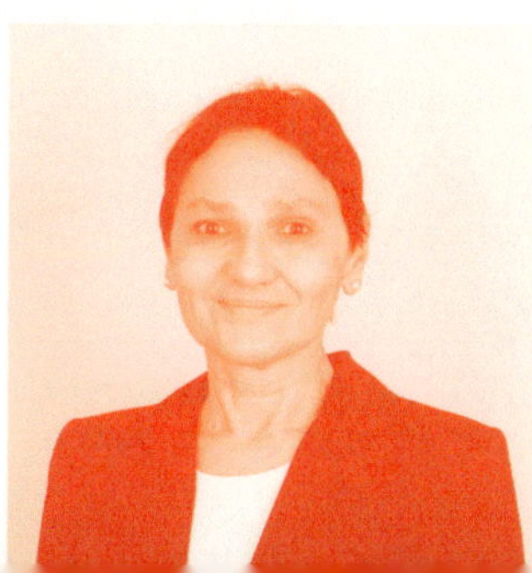

Molecular Pharmacology
http://dx.doi.org/10.5772/intechopen.89926
Edited by Angel Catala and Usama Ahmad

Contributors
Marilena Vlachou, Angeliki Siamidi, Dimitrios Rekkas, Eleni Tsintavi, Peeush Singhal, Rajneesh Dutt Kaushik, Vijay Jyoti Kumar, Radmila Novakovic, Arfaxad Reyes-Alcaraz, Akira Naito, Mani Sharma, Jyoti Joshi, Neeraj Kumar Chouhan, Mamta N Talati, Sandeep Vaidya, Abhiram Kumar, Chad Brenner, Nicole Michmerhuizen, Jiayu Wang, Usama Ahmad, Asad Ali, Zeeshan Ahmad, Mohd Muazzam Khan, Md. Faheem Haider, Juber Akhtar, Emilio Y. Lucero Garcia-Rojas, Richard A. Bond, Bradley K. McConnell, Vladimir Djokic

First published in London, United Kingdom, 2021 by IntechOpen
IntechOpen is the global imprint of INTECHOPEN LIMITED, registered in England and Wales, registration number: 11086078, 5 Princes Gate Court, London, SW7 2QJ, United Kingdom
Printed in Croatia

British Library Cataloguing-in-Publication Data
A catalogue record for this book is available from the British Library

Additional hard and PDF copies can be obtained from orders@intechopen.com

Molecular Pharmacology
Edited by Angel Catala and Usama Ahmad
p. cm.
Print ISBN 978-1-83962-931-0
Online ISBN 978-1-83962-932-7
eBook (PDF) ISBN 978-1-83962-933-4

For EU product safety concerns:
IN TECH d.o.o., Prolaz Marije Krucifikse Kozulić 3, 51000 Rijeka, Croatia, info@intechopen.com or visit our website at intechopen.com.

Meet the editors

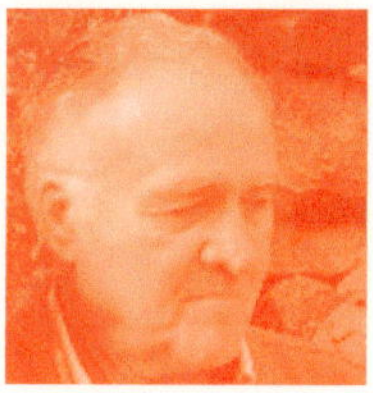

Angel Catalá was born in Rodeo (San Juan, Argentina). He studied chemistry at Universidad Nacional de La Plata, Argentina, where he received a PhD in Chemistry (Biological Branch) in 1965. From 1964 to 1974, he worked as Assistant in Biochemistry at the School of Medicine at the same university. From 1974 to 1976, he was a fellow of the National Institutes of Health (NIH) at the University of Connecticut, Health Center, USA. From 1985 to 2004, he served as Full Professor of Biochemistry at the Universidad Nacional de La Plata. He is a member of the National Research Council (CONICET), Argentina, and Argentine Society for Biochemistry and Molecular Biology (SAIB). His laboratory has been interested for many years in the lipid peroxidation of biological membranes from various tissues and different species. Dr. Catalá has directed twelve doctoral theses, published more than 100 papers in peer-reviewed journals, several chapters in books, and edited twelve books. He received awards at the 40th International Conference Biochemistry of Lipids 1999 in Dijon (France). He is winner of the Bimbo Pan-American Nutrition, Food Science and Technology Award 2006 and 2012, South America, Human Nutrition, Professional Category. In 2006, he won the Bernardo Houssay award in pharmacology, in recognition of his meritorious works of research. Dr. Catalá belongs to the editorial board of several journals including *Journal of Lipids*; *International Review of Biophysical Chemistry*; *Frontiers in Membrane Physiology and Biophysics*; *World Journal of Experimental Medicine and Biochemistry Research International*; *World Journal of Biological Chemistry, Diabetes and the Pancreas; International Journal of Chronic Diseases & Therapy*; and *International Journal of Nutrition*. He is the co-Editor of *The Open Biology Journal* and associate Editor for *Oxidative Medicine and Cellular Longevity*.

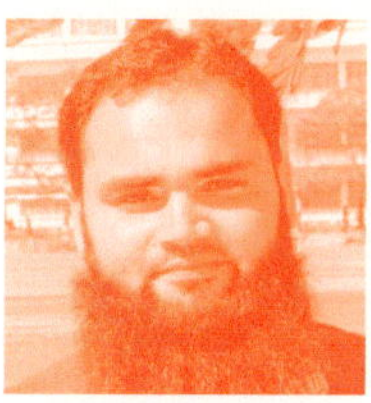

Dr. Usama Ahmad holds a specialization in Pharmaceutics from Amity University, Lucknow, India. He received his Ph.D. degree from the Integral University on his work titled 'Development and evaluation of silymarin nanoformulation for hepatic carcinoma'. Currently, he's working as an Assistant Professor of Pharmaceutics in the Faculty of Pharmacy, Integral University. He has been teaching Pharm.D, B.Pharm, and M.Pharm students and conducting research in the novel drug delivery domain. From 2013 to 2014 he worked on a research project funded by SERB-DST, Government of India. He has a rich publication record with more than 17 original articles published in reputed journals, 1 edited book with IntechOpen, 2 book chapters (1 with McGraw Hill Publishers and other with IntechOpen), and a number of scientific articles published in 'Ingredients South Asia Magazine' and 'QualPharma Magazine'. He is a member of the American Association for Cancer Research, Commonwealth Pharmacist Association, and the British Society for Nanomedicine. Dr. Ahmad's research focus is on the development of nanoformulations to facilitate the delivery of drugs that aim to provide practical solutions to current healthcare problems.

Contents

Preface

Molecular pharmacology has received increased attention in recent years. Nevertheless, due to its various forms and applications, the field requires further investigation.

This book covers topics ranging from the application of original structural biology, biochemistry, biophysics, physiology, genetics, and molecular biology to basic problems significant for the field of pharmacology. Chapters are contributions by invited researchers with long-standing experience in different research areas. We hope that the material presented here is understandable to a broad audience, including not only scientists but also people with a general background in the biological sciences. This volume offers up-to-date, expert reviews of the fast-moving field of pharmacology. The book is divided into three sections: Drug Transport, Pharmaceutical Dosage Forms and Structure of Drug-Receptor Complex.

The first section contains two chapters on:

1. "Liposome-A Comprehensive Approach for Researchers"

2. "Preparation and *in vitro* Characterisation of Solid Dispersion Floating Tablet by Effervescent Control Release Technique with Improved Floating Capabilities"

The second section contains one chapter on:

1. "3D-Printed Modified-Release Tablets: A Review of the Recent Advances"

The third section contains five chapters on:

1. "Integrated Molecular Profiling as an Approach to Identify PI3K Inhibitor Resistance Mechanisms"

2. "Allosteric Modulators for GPCRs as a Therapeutic Alternative with High Potential in Drug Discovery"

3. "Potassium Channels as a Potential Target Spot for Drugs"

4. "Fibril Formation by Glucagon in Solution and in Membrane Environments"

5. "Integrating Nanotherapeutic Platforms to Image Guided Approaches for Management of Cancer"

I would like to express my gratitude to Publishing Process Manager Jasna Božić and IntechOpen for their efforts in the publishing process.

Angel Català
Facultad de Ciencias Exactas,
Instituto de Investigaciones Fisicoquímicas Teóricas y Aplicadas
(INIFTA-CCT La Plata-CONICET),
Universidad Nacional de La Plata,
La Plata, Argentina

Usama Ahmad
Integral University,
India

Section 1

Drug Transport

Chapter 1

Liposome-A Comprehensive Approach for Researchers

Mani Sharma, Jyoti Joshi, Neeraj Kumar Chouhan, Mamta N. Talati, Sandeep Vaidya and Abhiram Kumar

Abstract

Bangham was first to develop these spherical-shaped nano-vesicles called liposomes in the early 1960s. Today, liposomes have emerged as crucial tools for bettering the delivery of drugs that majorly includes-antifungal drug, peptide hormones, enzymes, vaccines antimicrobial agents, drugs against cancer, and genetic materials. Following the different manufacturing practices and versatile properties liposomes can be categorized in various parameters of size, charge, poly-dispersity index, encapsulation efficiency, solubility properties, and lamellarity. Alteration in such parameters elevates the loading and bioavailability of a drug by giving more clear target specification, desired or controlled release. This bibliographic chapter provides a comprehensive overview of methods for the preparation of liposomes with other perspectives that majorly includes—physio-chemical characteristics, dosage regimen, advantages over other delivery systems, approved liposomal based drugs and other ongoing drugs in clinical trials. It will help researchers to break-through more structurally successful delivery vehicles depending upon their various physic-chemical properties.

Keywords: liposomes, particle size, zeta potential, polydispersity index, encapsulation efficiency, methods of preparation and bioavailability

1. Introduction

Liposomes can be microscopically examined as the vesicle with spherical structure that comprises one or more bilayer lipid in the aqueous core part of a shell. Liposomes are widely used in the delivery of variety of drugs depending upon its various physic-chemical characteristics. Design and development of liposomes are classified in many ways among which thin film hydration method is the most globally accepted procedure. Liposmes formation occurs when lipids are incorporated into water or buffer solution under continuous stirring, that in return forms the spherically shaped vesicles termed as liposomes. There are many methods to develop liposomes among which thin film hydration method is most common. Recently, lipid film hydration method was used to develop a multilamellar vesicle (MLV) loaded with curcumin (CUR) and Rhodamine B (RhB), [1] as a successful drug delivery approach. Phospholipids and cholesterol are the major components used in the development of liposomes (**Figure 1**). Where bilayer lipid composes of a hydrophilic head group, i.e., phospholipid and a hydrophilic tail group. Where phospholipids can easily penetrate and localize in the skin thus increases the overall

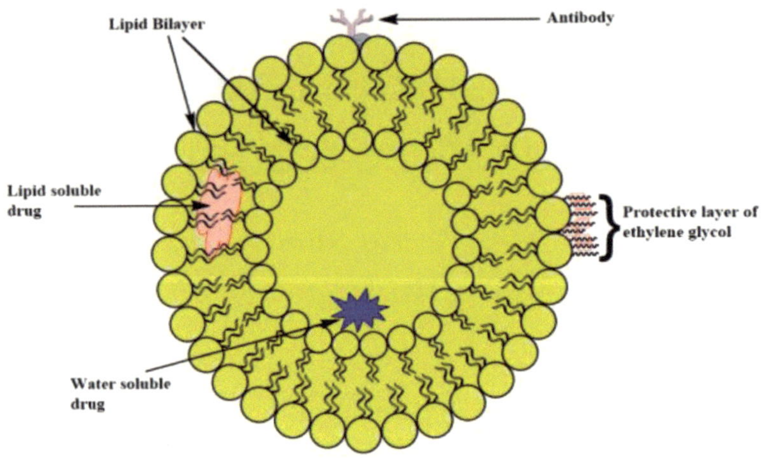

Figure 1.
Liposome molecule with lipid bilayer.

bioavailability in case of many dermal formulations whereas, cholesterol not only increases microviscosity of the bilayer but also defines the stability and rigidity of the formulation [2].

There are many routes to administer liposomes containing drugs, i.e., pulmonary, ocular, intramuscular, intravenous, topical, nasal and oral. Liposomes can be delivered in many ways involving sprays, capsules, ointments, creams, solutions, etc. for curing various disseases: bacterial, fungal, ocular, vaccines, fibrinolysis, endocrine, arthritis, asthma, diabetes, diseases of immune system, herpes, analgesics, topical anesthesia and even cancer [3].

Based on different parameters, liposomes are further classified depending upon method of preparation, structural parameters, biochemistry, cosmetics and medicine composition, and application in biology. Phospholipids can be from natural sources such as soya bean, egg yolk and olive oil. Depending upon various characteristics liposomes can be categorized on the basis of various physical parameters such as—pH, temperature, ionic charges, immunogenicity and stability.

In a recent study performed in 2019, it is revealed that the concentration of phospholipids and cholesterol variates the protein binding of the formulation [4].

Most commonly employed phospholipids in the formulation of liposomes are: phosphatidylserine (PS), phosphatidylcholine (PC), phosphatidylinositol (PI), phosphatidylethanolamine (PE), dipalmitoyl phosphatidylserine1,2dioleoylsnglycero3phosphoserine, dipalmitoylphosphatidylcholine (DPPC), distearoylphosphatidylcholine (DSPC), dioleoylphosphatidylethanolamine (DOPE) [5].

1.1 Composition of liposomes

A. Phospholipids

1. Derived from natural sources:

- Phosphatidylcholine
- Phosphatidylserine
- Phosphatidylethanolamine

2. Synthetic phospholipids:

    - Disloyal phosphatidylethanolamine

    - Disloyal phosphatidylcholine

B. Cholesterol

Cholesterol are optimized to be used in the formulation of liposomes up to a wide range with a molar ratios 1:1 or 2:1 against phospholipids. Cholesterol defines a strategic role in liposome composition; although, the adequate quantity to be used in the formulation has not been yet clarified. Thus, we can optimize lipids and cholesterol ratio, to prepare stable and controlled drug release vehicles (**Figures 2** and 3) [6].

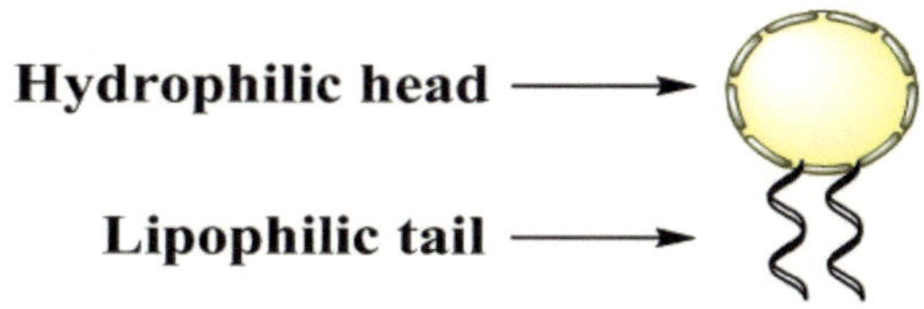

Figure 2.
Hydrophilic and lipophilic terminals of lipid.

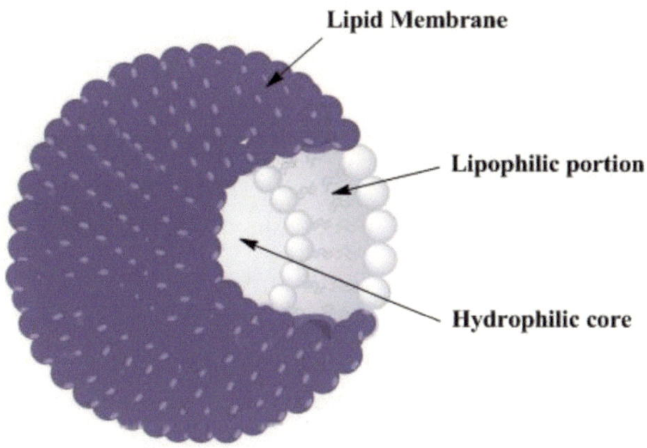

Figure 3.
Inner and outer structure of liposome.

2. Physio-chemical properties

See **Tables 1–3**.

3. Applications of liposomes

Role of liposome in drug delivery:

- Selective & passive targeting.

- It increases the overall therapeutic index and efficacy of a liposomal formulation.

Characterization parameters	Analytical method/instrument
Mean vesicle size and size distribution (submicron and micron range)	Zetasizer
Vesicle shape and surface morphology	Transmission electron microscopy
Electrical surface potential and surface pH	Zetasizer & pH measurement device
Surface charge free	Flow electrophoresis
Phase behavior	Differential scanning calorimetry (DSC)
Lamellarity	Freeze-fracture electron microscopy
Percent of free drug/percent capture	Minicolumn centrifugation, ion-exchange chromatography, radiolabelling

Table 1.
Physical characterization [6].

Characterization parameters	Analytical method/instrument
Phospholipid concentration	Barlett assay, Stewart assay, HPLC
Concentration of cholesterol	By HPLC
Phopholipid peroxidation	UV absorbance, iodometric, GLC

Table 2.
Chemical characterization [6].

Characterization parameters	Analytical method/instrument
Sterility aerobic or anaerobic cultures	Sterility aerobic or anaerobic cultures
Pyrogenicity	Limulus amebocyte lysate (LAL) test
Animal toxicity	By pathology and histology

Table 3.
Biological characterization [6].

- Due to the encapsulation of drug, overall stability is increased and reduced the adverse effects of encapsulated drug.

- It helps to improve the pharmacokinetic processes by increasing the circulation lifetime, decreasing elimination and toxic effects thus elevating the overall bioavailability of a drug [7].

- Active targeting can also be achieved by coupling with the site-specific ligands.

3.1 Other advantages of using liposomes

- Biodegradability

- Efficient control of the release

- Resemblance to natural membrane structures

- Increased targeting prospects

- Biocompatibility
- Biodegradable
- Liposomes are able to provide both aqueous "milieu internee" and the lipophilic environment in a single system
- It helps in protecting the encapsulated drug.
- Method of preparation is easy and has no such complicated or expensive procedures involved
- Facilitates both active and passive targeting.
- No toxicity in heart as it does not accumulates in the heart.
- Intercepts the oxidation of drug
- Chelation therapy in case of of heavy metal poisoning
- Diagnostic imaging of tumors
- In enzyme replacement therapy
- Study of membranes
- In gene delivery
- As drug delivery carriers
- In multidrug resistance
- In immunology
- In cosmetology (**Table 4**)

Category	**Application utilized**
In parasitic diseases	After IV injection liposomes are comfortly digested by phagocytic cells in the body and hence considered as one of the best vehicle to dispatch cargo into macrophages
Anticancer therapy	Liposomes are effective for the cells not only in tumors but also in the gastrointestinal mucosa
Other medical applications	These liposomes are sterically stabilized vesicles and are long circulating micro-reservoirs or tumor (or site of inflammation and infection) targeting vehicles
In bioengineering	Fragments of siRNA and DNA are delivered with the help of modern genetic engineering and gene recombinant technology
In vaccination	Liposomes are considerably used in proper vaccination due its fine active targeting
In agro-food industry	Due to its versatile physio-chemical properties lipids are extensively manufactured and used in large scale up sectors

Table 4.
Applications of liposomes [6].

4. Methods of preparation

See **Figure 4**.

4.1 Thin film hydration method

This is one of the widely used methods for the preparation of liposomes. As it has no such complicated steps involved in it. Multilamellar vesicles (MLV) are prepared by solubilizing natural or synthesized phospholipid in chloroform, dichloromethane, ethanol or in a mixture of chloroform and methanol in a ratio of 3:1 v/v; 2:1 v/v or 9:1 v/v. A homogeneous thin film forms when this mixture is revolved and dried in a rota-evaporator under vacuum at a temperature around 45–60°C. Layes is kept under nitrogen drying for overnight. Next, comes the hydration process where completely dried thin film is hydrated using aqueous phase—phosphate buffer solution of pH 7.2 for 1–2 h at 60–70°C.

This kind of procedure can be applied to almost any kind of lipid mixtures, but has some drawbacks that majorly includes—low encapsulation space, a bit difficult to scale up and layer formed are not always homogeneous thus shows heterogeneous size distribution during later physio-chemical examination of liposomes through zetasizer.

4.2 Injection methods

4.2.1 Ether injection method

Here, the lipid mixture is dissolved in ether or diethyl ether under continuous stirring that is later injected into a PBS or aqueous phase. Which under injection pressure causes the removal of almost all organic solvent that ultimately forms liposomes. This method also suffers with the heterogeneous liposomal formulation defect.

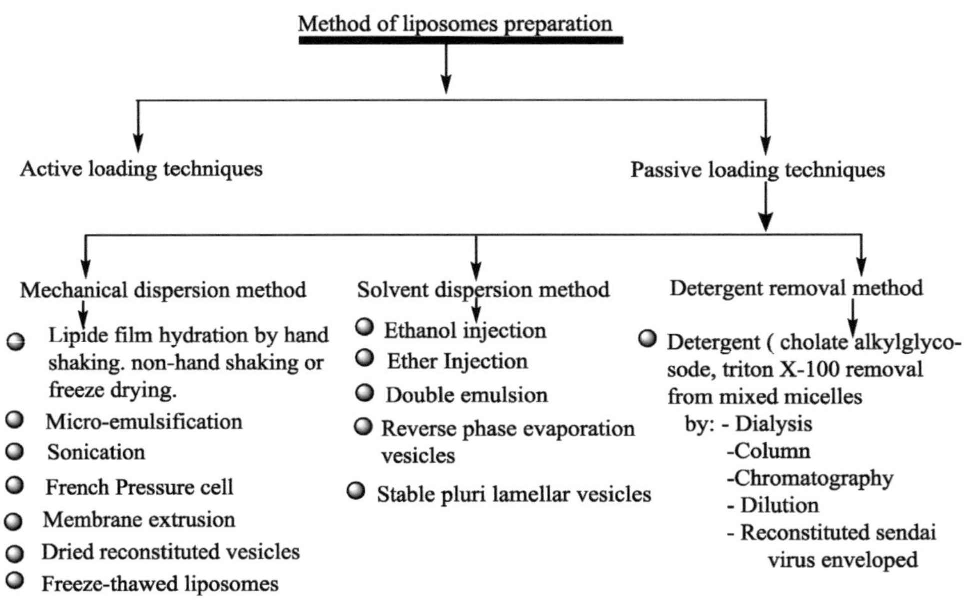

Figure 4.
General representation for method of preparation of liposome.

4.2.2 Ethanol injection method

In ethanol injection method the lipid mixture is dissolved in ethanol under continuous stirring that is later injected into a preheated TRIS-HCl buffer or distilled water. Hydrophobicity and hydrophilicity of a drug accounts for drug intake in a liposomal vesicle. It has an advantage of using non-toxic and ethanol and is also easily scalable.

4.3 Sonication method

It is the most widely accepted method to develop small unilamellar vesicles (SLV). SLV are prepared by solubilizing natural or synthesized phospholipid in chloroform, dichloromethane, ethanol or in a mixture of chloroform and methanol in a ratio of 3:1 v/v; 2:1 v/v or 9:1 v/v. A homogeneous thin film forms when this mixture is revolved and dried in a rota-evaporator under vaccum at a temperature around 45–60°C. Layes is kept under nitrogen drying for overnight. Next, comes the hydration process where completely dried thin film is hydrated using aquous phase—phosphate buffer solution of pH 7.2 for 1–2 h at 60–70°C. Further the bath sonicator is used to transform the size of vesicles. Lastly, liposomes are centrifuged in order to remove the titanium particles that might got added due to overheating in sonication process. Less encapsulation space is the major drawback of such vesicles.

4.4 High-pressure extrusion method

Liposomes are prepared by solubilizing natural or synthesized phospholipid in chloroform, dichloromethane, ethanol or in a mixture of chloroform and methanol in a ratio of 3:1 v/v; 2:1 v/v or 9:1 v/v. A homogeneous thin film forms when this mixture is revolved and dried in a rota-evaporator under vacuum at a temperature around 45–60°C. Layes is kept under nitrogen drying for overnight. Next, comes the hydration process where completely dried thin film is hydrated using aqueous phase—phosphate buffer solution of pH 7.2 for 1–2 h at 60–70°C. In addition, these lipoosmes are passes through high pressure extruder for 10 cycles in order to obtain more uniform and stable liposomes.

4.5 Reverse-phase evaporation method

Here, the lipid mixture is dissolved in organic solvents ether or diethyl ether or a mixture of diethyl ether and chloroform (1:1 v/v); a mixture of methanol-chloroform (1:2 v/v) under continuous stirring that is later injected into a PBS or aqueous phase comprising citric-Na_2HPO_4 to improve the overall efficacy of a formulation. Which under injection pressure causes the removal of organic solvent that ultimately leads to the formation of liposomes. This method also suffers with the heterogeneous liposomal formulation defect. Organic solvent is then dried using rota-vapor instrument thus forming homogeneous liposome. The major disadvantage of this procedure is the leftover of remaining organic solvent in the final formulation also faces difficulty in scale up procedures.

4.6 Calcium-induced fusion method

Here acidic phospholipids are used to prepare SUV by following the thin film hydration process followed on with the addition of calcium that causes fusion to form MLV. Final addition of ethylenediaminetetraacetic acid (EDTA) to MLV results in the formation of large unilamellar vesicles LUV.

4.7 Dehydration-rehydration method

Liposomes are prepared by using the sonication method as explained in Section 4.3. Developed liposomes are freeze dried overnight where the formation of multi-lamellar vesicles occurs when dry powder gets controlled rehydration.

4.8 Freeze-thaw method

Liposomes are prepared by using thin film hydration method as explained in Section 4.1. Developed liposomes are freeze dried overnight and is then thawed

Drugs liposome formulation	Method	Type of liposome
Antifungal drugs		
Amphotericin B	Thin-film hydration method	MLV
Clotrimazole	Rotary evaporation method	MLV
Fluconazole	Thin film hydration method	MLV
Analgesic drugs		
Ketorolac tromethamine	Thin-film hydration method	MLV
Antibiotic drugs		
Amikacin	Reverse phase evaporation method	MLV, LUV
Mafenide acetate	Solvent evaporation and microencapsulation	MLV SUV
Antifibrinolytic drugs		
Tranexamic acid	Chloroform film and sonication method	SUV
Drugs against cancer		
5-Fluorouracil	Lipid-film hydration method, extrusion, ethanol injection and reverse phase evaporation method	MLV, LUV, SUV MLV, LUV
Vinblastine sulphate	Thin-film hydration method and sonication	MLV SUV
Tamoxifen	Thin-film hydration method	MLV
Bis-demethoxy curcumin analogue	Thin-film hydration method and sonication	MLV SUV
Doxorubicin	Lipid-film hydration method and extrusion	MLV
Hormone drugs		
Cyproterone acetate	Thin-film hydration method	MLV
Immunosuppressive drugs		
Sirolimus	Thin-film hydration method	MLV
Tacrolimus (Fk-506)	Thin-film hydration method	MLV
Ophthalmic drugs		
Brimonidine tartrate	Thin-film hydration method and sonication	MLV SUV
Acetazolamide	Reverse phase evaporation and thin-film hydration method	MLV, LUV MLV
Potential drugs as oral insulin		
Sodium glycocholate and metformin hydrochloride	Reverse phase evaporation and thin-film hydration method	MLV, LUV MLV
Vaccines		
Tetanus toxoid diphtheria toxoid	Reverse phase evaporation method	MLV, LUV

Table 5.
Methods for the preparation of liposomal formulation to deliver drugs [2].

in order to govern the ionic strength and phospholipid concentration of the final liposomal formation. Physical disruption of lamellar structure occurs due to freeze-thaw of liposomal formulation giving it a final ionic structure.

4.9 Microfluidization

Boltic et al. was the first to introduce such method for the preparation of liposomes. Here liposomes are prepared using thin film hydration method as explained in Section 4.1, which is then sonicated and microfluidized in order to obtain partial homogenization. This method has its wide application in industrial formulation of liposomes.

4.10 Supercritical fluids (SCF)

Supercritical fluids (SCF) were introduced to replace toxic organic solvents for the preparation of liposomes. Supercritical carbon dioxide is the most widely used supercritical fluid as it has many advantages over conventionally used organic solvents such as—it is not flammable, can be recycled, non-toxic, can be comparatively easily removed from the solvents, requires moderate temperature and also exclude the product degradation in inert surroundings. Karn et al. experimented and explained the comparative study between thin film hydration method and supercritical fluids using method evaluating the non toxicity and better field approaches in term of using super critical fluids for the formulation of liposomes (**Table 5**).

5. Mechanism of liposomal formulation

- Phospholipids shows affinity for polar molecules as well as for **aqueous** phase due to a hydrophobic tail, that has 2 fatty acids which are made up of 10–24 C atoms comprising of 0–6 double bonds in every chain [8].

- In a phospholipid molecule the polar portion connects with a polar environment of a aqueous medium.

- Phospholipids arrange layers of lipids in close alignment in a planer bilayer sheet. Sufficient amount of energy is required for this planar arrangement (sonication, homogenization, heating, etc.) (**Figure 5**).

6. Evaluation

6.1 Morphological and physicochemical characterization of liposomal-formulation

The average size, size distribution, and zeta potential shall be determined by zetasizer.

Transmission electron microscopy is used to study the shape and surface morphology of a liposomal structure.

6.2 In vitro performance evaluation and stability studies

Stability studies: stability studies shall be conducted to assess the shelf-life of product as per ICH guidelines.

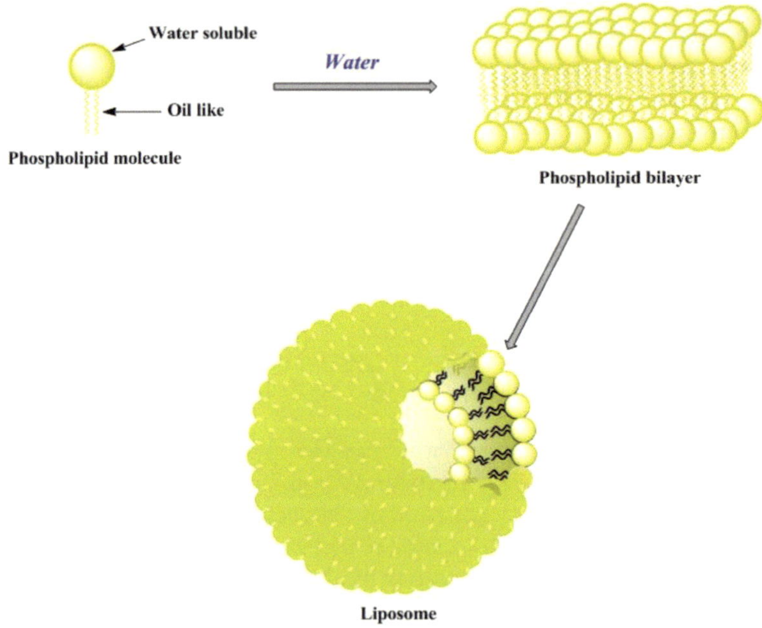

Figure 5.
Mechanism of liposome formation.

MTT [3-(4,5-dimethythiazol-2-yl)-2,5-diphenyl tetrazolium bromide] assay to evaluate the in-vitro cytotoxicity of the developed formulation.

FACS (fluorescence assisted cell sorting) is used to quantify the cell uptake study.

7. Marketed liposomal formulations

See **Tables 6** and 7.

Marketed product	Drug used	Target diseases	Company
Alec™	Dry protein free powder of DPPC PG	Expanding lung diseases in babies	Britannia Pharm, UK
Ventus™	Prostaglandin E1	Systemic inflammatory diseases	The liposome company, USA
Topex Br	Terbutaline sulphate	Asthma ozone	USA
Doxil™ or Caelyx™	Doxorubicin	Kaposi's sarcoma	SEQUUS, USA
Novasome	Smallpox vaccine	Smallpox	Novavax USA
Evacet™ Doxorubicin	Doxorubicin	Metastatic breast cancer	The Liposome Company, USA
Fungizone®	Amphotericin B	Fungal infections	Leishmaniasis
Depocyt	Cytarabine	Cancer therapy	Skye Pharm USA
Doxil®	Doxorubicin HCl	Refractory ovarian cancer	ALZA, USA

Marketed product	Drug used	Target diseases	Company
Amphotec™	Amphotericin	B fungal infections, leishmaniasis	SEQUUS, USA

Table 6.
Liposomal formulations present in the market [9].

Product	Manufacturer	Liposomes and key ingredients
Formule Liposome Gel	Formule Liposome Gel Payot (Ferdinand Muehlens)	(Thymoxin) hyaluronic acid
Symphatic 2000	Biopharm GmbH	Thymus extract vitamin A palmitate
Niosomes	Lancome (L'Or'eal)	Glyceropolyether with moisturizers
Inovita	Pharm/Apotheke	Thymus extract, hyaluronic
Future Perfect Skin Gel	Estee Lauder	TMF, Vitamins E, A palmitate, cerebroside ceramide
Flawless finish	Elizabeth Arden	Liquid make up
Eye Perfector	Avon	Soothing cream to reduce eye
Nactosomes	Lancome (L'Or'eal)	Vitamins
Efect du Soleil	L'Or'eal	Tanning agents in liposomes niosomes lancome
Natipide II	Nattermann PL	Liposomal gel for do-it yourself

Table 7.
Liposomal cosmetic formulations present in the market [10].

8. Conclusions

Liposomes evolved as an extraordinary tool or micro-engineered membranes for the delivery of drugs because of their minimum toxicity and flexibility that can be tailored for various desirable intentions. This unparalleled delivery approach can be used for almost every drug or active pharmaceutical ingredient despite of its varied physicochemical properties and route of administration. Extensive uses of liposome in the delivery of drugs can be starched further by researchers, medical representatives and in scale-up processes in order to develop desired modification and better delivery approaches by holding the promising physio-chemical properties and pharmacokinetics (absorption, distribution, metabolism, and elimination) involved with liposomes, as described in the chapter.

Acknowledgements

I thank all my coauthors who are listed, and the work was not funded by any institute or person.

Conflict of interest

We wish to declare that there are no known conflicts of interest associated with this publication, and there has been no significant financial support for this work that could have influenced its outcome.

Author details

Mani Sharma[1*], Jyoti Joshi[1], Neeraj Kumar Chouhan[2], Mamta N. Talati[2], Sandeep Vaidya[2] and Abhiram Kumar[1]

1 Uttarakhand Technical University [UKTU], Uttarakhand, India

2 National Institute of Pharmaceutical Education and Research [NIPER], Telangana, India

*Address all correspondence to: mninup2015@gmail.com

References

[1] Anishiya Chella ER, Rajendran NK, Jeyaraj M, Ramu A, Rajan M. Retinal photoreceptors targeting SA-g-AA coated multilamellar liposomes carrier system for cytotoxicity and cellular uptake evaluation. Journal of Liposome Research. 2020:1-35. ISSN: 0898-2104

[2] Popovska O. An overview: Methods for preparation and characterization of liposomes as drug delivery systems. International Journal of Pharmaceutical and Phytopharmacological Research. 2014;**3**(3):182-189

[3] Pandey RS. Formulation of benzocaine loaded PG-liposomes for enhanced skin delivery. Asian Journal of Medical and Pharmaceutical Sciences. 2012;**2**:78-82

[4] Foteini P, Pippa N, Naziris N, Demetzos C. Physicochemical study of the protein–liposome interactions: Influence of liposome composition and concentration on protein binding. Journal of Liposome Research. 2019;**29**(4):313-321

[5] Sharma SH, Mishra LI, Grover I, Gupta AN, Kaur KI. Liposomes: Vesicular system an overview. International Journal of Pharmacy and Pharmaceutical Sciences. 2010;**2**(4):15-21

[6] Dwivedi C, Verma S. Review on preparation and characterization of liposomes with application. Journal of Scientific and Innovative Research. 2013;**2**:486-508

[7] Sesarman A, Muntean D, Abrudan B, Tefas L, Sylvester B, Licarete E, et al. Improved pharmacokinetics and reduced side effects of doxorubicin therapy by liposomal co-encapsulation with curcumin. Journal of Liposome Research. 2019;**8**:1-10

[8] Unga J, Omata D, Kudo N, Ueno S, Munakata L, Shima T, et al. Development and evaluation of stability and ultrasound response of DSPC-DPSG-based freeze-dried microbubbles. Journal of Liposome Research. 2019;**29**(4):368-374

[9] Sackmann E. Physical basis of self-organization and function of membranes: Physics of vesicles. In: Handbook of Biological Physics. Vol. 1. 1995. pp. 213-304

[10] Lasic DD, Frederik PM, Stuart MC, Barenholz Y, McIntosh TJ. Gelation of liposome interior A novel method for drug encapsulation. FEBS Letters. 1992;**312**(2-3):255-258

Chapter 2

Preparation and *in vitro* Characterisation of Solid Dispersion Floating Tablet by Effervescent Control Release Technique with Improved Floating Capabilities

Peeush Singhal, Rajneesh Dutt Kaushik and Vijay Jyoti Kumar

Abstract

In this research, an effort has been done for the development of effervescent controlled release floating tablet (ECRFT) from solid dispersions (SDs) of diclofenac sodium (DS) for upsurge the solubility and dissolution rate. ECRFT of DS was prepared by using SDs of DS and its SDs prepared with PEG as carrier using thermal method (simple fusion). SDs of DS was formulated in many ratios (1:1, 1:2, 1:3 and 1:4). Prepared SDs were optimised for its solubility, % drug content and % dissolution studies. Tablets were formulated by using optimised SDs products and all formulation was evaluated for various parameters. A clear rise in dissolution rate was detected with entirely SD, amid that the optimised SD (SD4) was considered for ECRFT. Among all the tablet formulations, its F3 formulation was better in all the terms of pre-compression and post-compression parameters. It had all the qualities of a good ECRFT, based on this F3 formulation was selected as the best formulation. Data of *in vitro* release were fitted in several kinetics models to explain release mechanism. The F3 formulation shows zero order release. From this study, we can conclude that ECRFT containing SDs of DS can be successfully used for achieving better therapeutic objective.

Keywords: solid dispersion, diclofenac sodium, polyethylene glycol, dissolution enhancement, floating tablets

1. Introduction

Diclofenac sodium (DS) is an effective NSAID with high affinity for both COX-1 and COX-2 receptors and it is one and only maximum frequently recommended drugs in India for the cure of pain, inflammation and joint stiffness caused by arthritis. According to BCS classification system DS belonging from class II means to say having poor solubility and poor dissolution rate [1] hence the focus of this study was on converting BCS class from II to I by increasing its solubility and dissolution rate of DS Which was taken as model drug [2]. The release rate can be improved by increasing surface area of existing drug by using several techniques but among these methods solid dispersion technique is one of the best techniques for increasing the surface area [3]. Hence, an effort was made to increase the dissolution characteristics using the solid dispersion technique [3, 4]. It has absorption site in upper part of gastro intestinal tract. Gastric retention of DS was very short that is why the bioavailability of drug is 54% which is very low because near about 50% portion of orally given drug misses the absorption window. The pharmacokinetic profile of DS showed that the half-life is about ~1.2–2 h and hence there is a requirement of frequent dosing (3–4 tablets daily) [5] but this requirement of frequent dose is very dangerous for patients because due to this frequent dosing fluctuation in plasma drug level in body and need constant monitoring of patient for adjustment of dose regimen. That is why this reason may consequently support faster absorption of drug in stomach with higher concentrations for bioavailability improvement. Therefore in order to improve drug dissolution and reduced dosing frequency, it was attempted to formulate solid dispersion of DS [6, 7] and then develop effervescent controlled release floating tablet [8]. The emphasis of the current research was to increase the release rate and bioavailability of DS through preparing ECRFT (effervescent control release floating tablets) with dual approach [9] using solid dispersion product of DS in order to regulate the drug release and make available security from first pass metabolism.

2. Methodologies

2.1 Preformulation studies

Prior to the development of dosage forms, it is essential that certain fundamental, physical and chemical properties of the drug molecule and other derived properties of the drug powder are determined and should be considered in the formulation in relation to the proposed dosage form and route of administration.

These studies should focus on those physiochemical properties of the drug that could affect drug performance and development of an efficacious dosage form.

A typical preformulation program should begin with the description of the organoleptic qualities of the drug substance. The colour, odour and taste are of immense value in developing an aesthetically acceptable formulation.

2.1.1 Identification and characterisation of diclofenac sodium

2.1.1.1 Physical appearance

Drug sample has been noted for its organoleptic properties. The drug is white to slightly yellowish crystalline powder, odour: slight and characteristic [1]. Drug was received as gift sample (15 g) from Kwality Pharmaceuticals Ltd., Amritsar.

2.1.1.2 Melting point determination

The melting point of compound is the temperature at which it changes from a solid to liquid [10]. This is a physical property often used to identify compounds.

2.1.1.2.1 Procedure

a. A capillary melting tube was taken.

b. A small amount of compound was placed on a clean surface. The compound was put in to open end of capillary tube.

c. The capillary melting point tube was placed in melting point apparatus (Macro scientific works).The sample was observed continuously, so that the melting point of the sample was not missed. Slow heating was done for most accurate results. The melting range was recorded which beings when the sample first starts to melt and ends when the sample completely melted.

2.1.1.3 Solubility studies

Solubility may be defined as the spontaneous interaction of two or more substances to form a homogeneous dispersion [11]. The solubility of diclofenac sodium was studied in various aqueous and non-aqueous solvents. About 10 mg of drug was taken in 10 ml of each solvent at room temperature in screw-capped test tubes and shaken for 30 min in a sonicator. The solubility was checked by U-V spectroscopy in all cases and reported in **Table 1**.

2.1.1.4 U.V. spectrophotometer

The organic molecule in solution when exposed to light in the ultra-violet region of the spectrum, absorbed light of particular wavelength depending on the type of electronic transition associated with absorption [12].

2.1.1.4.1 Diclofenac sodium

The solution (10 μg) of diclofenac sodium was prepared in simulated gastric fluid pH 1.2 and scanned spectrophotometrically (Systronics, Double beam UV-VIS Spectrophotometer: 2201). The scanning range was in between 200 nm to 400 nm. Standard solution of diclofenac sodium was then scanned and graph plotted. The

Parameter	Evaluation
API	DICLOFENAC SODIUM
Description	Crystalline
Colour	White
Odour	Odourless
Bulk Density	0.56 gm/ml
True Density	0.64 gm/ml
Carr's Index	14.28%
Hausner's Ratio	1.14
Melting Point	STD: 280°C OBS: 282–283°C
Solubility	Sparingly soluble: Water Freely soluble: methanol Soluble: 0.1 N HCl Insoluble: ether, chloroform and toluene
Partition coefficient	1.25

Table 1.
Preformulation characters of diclofenac sodium.

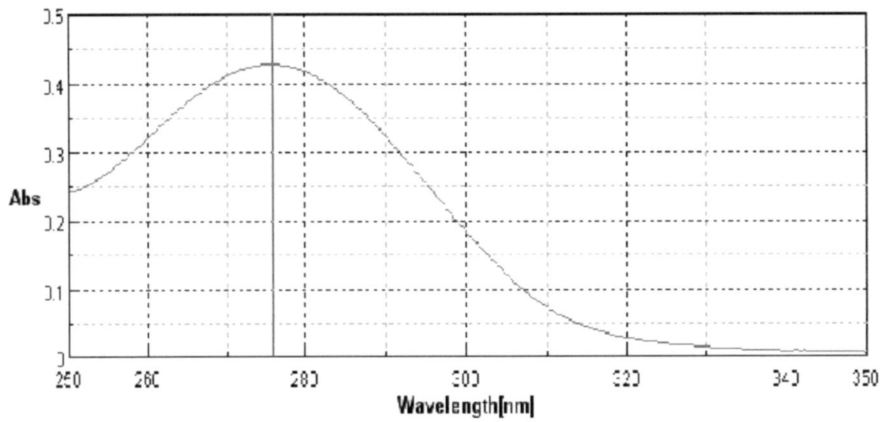

Figure 1.
U.V. scan of diclofenac sodium in simulated gastric fluid (PH 1.2).

determined λmax, 276 nm (**Figure 1**) was similar as reported in the literature (276 nm).

2.1.1.5 I.R. spectrophotometry

About 1 mg of the sample and 100 mg of the potassium bromide (KBr) was taken in a mortar and triturated [13]. A small amount of triturated sample was taken into a pellet maker and compressed at 10 kg/cm^2. The pellet was kept onto the sample holder and scanned from 4000 to 400 cm^{-1}.The I-R spectrum of drug sample was obtained using FTIR-8400 s, shimadzu. Important peaks are reported in **Table 2** and graphically represented in **Figures 2, 3**. This I-R spectrum was found concordant with the IR of diclofenac sodium reported in the official monograph.

2.1.1.6 Quantitative estimation of drug

For the present study the spectrophotometric method given in the official books was selected for its sensitivity, specificity, simplicity, reproducibility, rapidity and accuracy [14].

2.1.1.7 Preparation of calibration curve of diclofenc sodium in simulated gastric fluid (pH 1.2)

Accurately weighed 50 mg of drug (diclofenac sodium) was dissolved in 100 ml of simulated gastric fluid pH 1.2 to give a solution of 500 μg/ml concentration and

IR spectrum	Standard peaks value	Observed peaks value cm^{-1}	Groups	Stretching/ deformation
DICLOFENC SODIUM	1600–1475	1556.61, 1498.74	C=C(aromatic)	Stretching
	1320–1210	1305.85	C—O stretching	Stretching
	1556	1556.61	Dichlorophenyl ring	Stretching
	1300–1000	1284.63	C—CO—C stretching	Stretching

Table 2.
Characteristic peaks of diclofenac sodium.

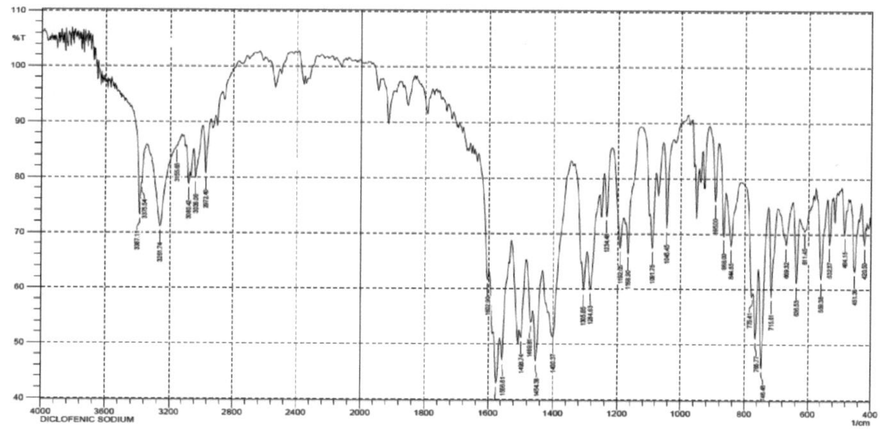

Figure 2.
FTIR spectroscopy of pure diclofenac sodium.

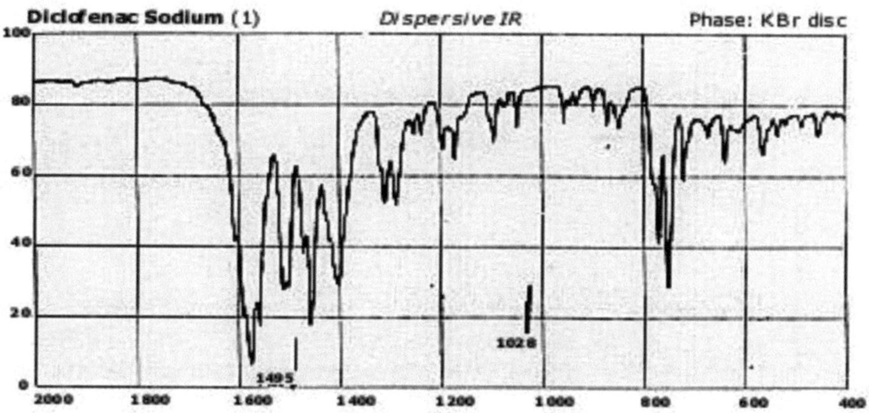

Figure 3.
I-R spectra of pure diclofenac sodium from I.P. 1996.

this was served as a standard solution [15, 16]. From this solution 10 ml was taken and diluted to 100 ml using simulated gastric fluid pH 1.2 to get a solution of 50 μg/ml concentration and this solution was served as the standard solution. In to a series of 10 ml volumetric flasks, aliquots of standard solution (i.e. 0.4, 0.8, 1.2, 1.6, 2.0, 3.0, 4.0, 5.0, 6.0 ml) were added and made up the volume up to 10 ml using simulated gastric fluid pH 1.2. The absorbance of these solutions was measured against reagent blank at 276 nm (**Table 3**). A standard curve between concentration and absorbance was plotted (**Figure 4**). A straight line passing through origin is obtained.

2.1.1.8 Partition coefficient

The partition coefficient directly influences the permeability of drug through various membranes [17–19]. The study has been designed to determine partition coefficient of drug in 1-octanol and pH 1.2 solutions. The partition coefficient between 1-octanol and Simulated gastric fluid (pH 1.2) was determined by shake flask method. About 10 mg of drug was dissolved in one of the phases, and is shaken with the other partitioning solvent for 30 min, allowed to stand for 5 min and then majority of the lower aqueous phase was run off. The drug concentration in both the

S. No	Concentration (µg/ml)	Abs(λmax-276 nm) (mean ± SD)
1	0	0.000 ± 0.00
2	2	0.068 ± 0.002
3	4	0.128 ± 0.005
4	6	0.190 ± 0.0015
5	8	0.246 ± 0.0021
6	10	0.315 ± 0.0022
7	12	0.329 ± 0.004
8	14	0.401 ± 0.001
9	16	0.445 ± 0.0032
10	18	0.522 ± 0.0051
11	20	0.589 ± 0.0059

Table 3.
Data for calibration curve of diclofenc sodium in simulated gastric fluid pH 1.2 at 276 nm (n = 3).

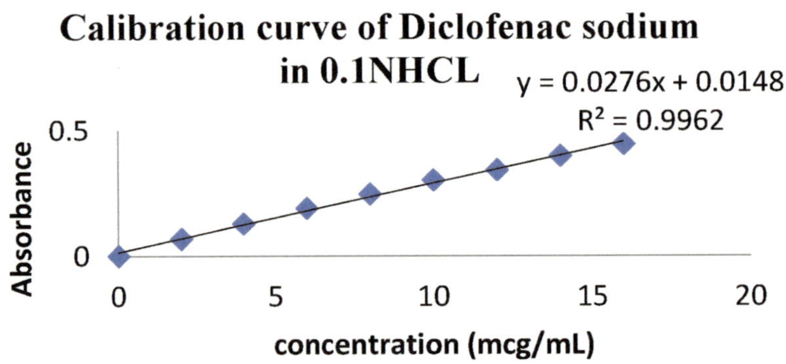

Figure 4.
Calibration curve of diclofenac sodium in pH 1.2 at 276 nm.

aqueous and 1-octanol phases was determined spectrophotometrically at 276 nm and calculated the partition coefficient. The partition coefficient was found to be 1.25.

$$\text{Partition Coefficient} = \text{Conc.of drug in oil phase}/\text{Conc.of drug in aqueous phase} \quad (1)$$

2.1.2 Result and discussion

Samples of diclofenac sodium obtained as a gift sample from kwality pharmaceuticals pvt. Ltd., Amritsar was identified and characterised as per the identification test given in official monograph. Physical appearance and melting point of the drug sample under investigation was found to be same as that of the official reports. The results are given in **Table 4**. The solubility of diclofenac sodium was determined in aqueous and non-aqueous solvents. Diclofenac sodium was found to be soluble in 0.1NHCl and ethanol; sparingly soluble in water, practically insoluble in ether, chloroform and toluene. Partition coefficient of the drug was found to be 1.25.The results are given in **Table 1**.

S. No	Melting ranges	Melting point (mean ± SD)
1	288–290°C	289.12 ± 0.21

Table 4.
Melting point result of diclofenac sodium.

The drug was identified by IR spectroscopy and the characteristic peaks obtained (**Figure 2**) compared with standard spectra (**Figure 3**) of pure drug reported in official monograph (IP1996). The IR spectra of drug sample are in agreement with the standard IR spectra of pure diclofenac sodium given in official monograph [1]. Important peaks are reported in **Table 2**.

In the present study, a reported U-V spectrophometric method was used for the estimation of diclofenac sodium. The calibration curve of diclofenac sodium was prepared in simulated gastric fluid pH 1.2. The data was regressed to obtain straight line. The correlation coefficient was found to be 0.996 in simulated gastric fluid pH 1.2 indicating good linearity. The calibration curve was found to obey Beer-Lamberts Law in the concentration range studied (0–20 μg/ml).

3. Materials

Diclofenac Sodium (Batch no. A5/206), hydroxyl propyl methyl cellulose (HPMC) K100M (Batch no. HP121406 MC) and crosspovidone (Batch no. YPVPP09319040) were obtained from kwality pharmaceutical pvt ltd Amritsar, as gift samples. Sodium bicarbonate (NaHCO3), citric acid, polyvinyl pyrrolidone (PVP K-30), magnesium stearate, lactose and Isopropyl alcohol were purchased from local suppliers. Marketed product, "Voveran SR100 or Voveran 50", (Manufactured by Ranbaxy, India; Batch no.131003 AU or 320,028), used for comparative studies, was purchased from the local retail pharmacy.

4. Methods

4.1 Preparation of physical mixtures (PM)

Physical mixtures were prepared by mixing the appropriate amounts of the drug and carrier (PEG 6000) in the different weight ratios of 1:1, 1:2, 1:3 and 1:4 in mortar [3, 4, 6, 7]. The resulting mixtures were sieved through sieve no. 80, collected and stored in closed container away from light and humidity until use.

4.2 Preparation of solid dispersion

Melt method was used to prepare solid dispersions of diclofenac sodium with PEG 6000 containing different weight ratio (1:1, 1:2, 1:3, 1:4, and 1:5) (**Table 5**). Diclofenac sodium and PEG 6000 were weighed according to their weighed ratios. PEG 6000 was melted at 60°C. In this melted PEG 6000, diclofenac sodium was added. It was mixed well and flashed cooled on an ice bath and then stored overnight in desiccators. The prepared solid dispersion was then grounded by using a mortar and pestle, sieved through a mesh no. 40 and stored over a fused calcium chloride in a desiccators' for further use.

S. no.	Ratio (diclofenac sodium:PEG6000)	Batch code
1	1:1	SD1
2	1:2	SD2
3	1:3	SD3
4	1:4	SD4
5	1:5	SD5

Table 5.
Composition of solid dispersion and there assign batch code.

4.3 Characterisation of solid dispersion/ physical mixtures of diclofenac sodium with PEG-6000SDs

4.3.1 FTIR spectroscopy

FTIR spectra of drug, PEG 6000 and solid dispersion of DS were obtained. About 1 mg of sample was mixed thoroughly with 100 mg potassium bromide IR powder and compacted under vacuum at a pressure of about 12 psi for 3 min. The resultant disc was mounted in a suitable holder in perkin elmer USA spectrum 65 IR spectrophotometer and the IR spectrum was recorded from 4000 to 400 cm^{-1} in a scan time of 12 min [20]. The resultant spectra were compared for any spectral changes. **Figure 5** shows the FTIR spectra of the (i) drug, (ii) carrier and (iii) Surface solid dispersion. There was no significant change in the spectrum of solid dispersions, as incorporation of diclofenac into the carrier (PEG6000) did not modify the position of its functional groups.

4.3.2 Determination of saturation solubility

Saturation solubility was determined by using shake flask method [20]. Excess quantities of pure DS, prepared SDs and PMs were added in 25 ml distilled water in

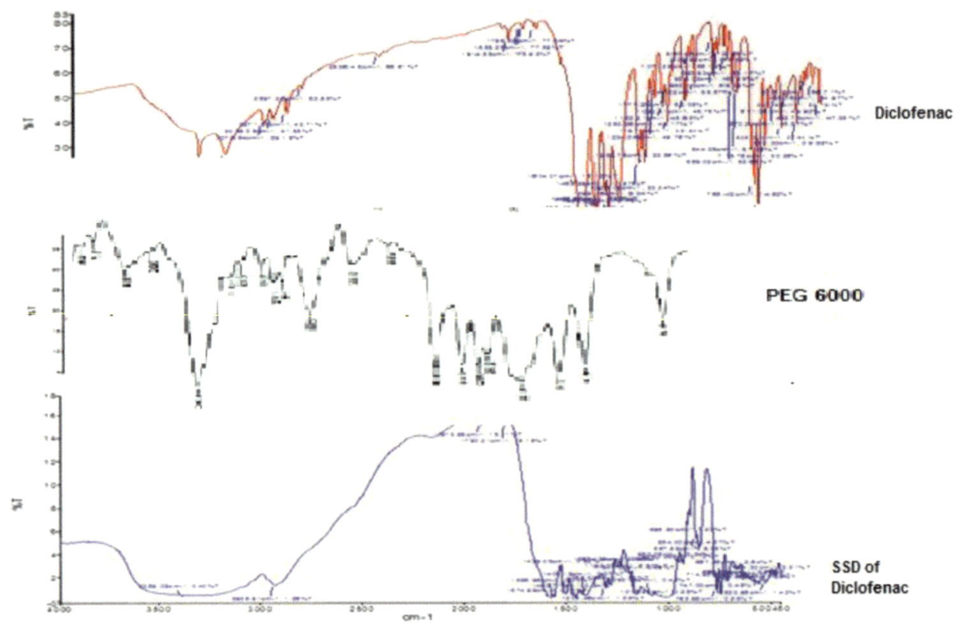

Figure 5.
Comparative FTIR spectra of diclofenac, PEG6000, & solid dispersion of diclofenac with PEG6000.

conical flasks which were then put in orbital shaker at 37°C and at 100 rpm for 72 h. Absorbance of resulting solution was measured on UV/Visible spectrophotometer (UV-1800 Shimadzu, Japan) at 276 nm.

4.3.3 Determination of pH dependent solubility

Shake flask method same as that for saturation solubility [20] was used with 0.1 N HCl.

4.3.4 Percent drug content

SDs equivalent to 50 mg of diclofenac sodium were weighed accurately and dissolved in 50 ml of ethanol by using mechanical shaker for 30 min. The solutions were filtered using whatman filter paper and drug content was determined by measuring absorbance at 276 nm by UV/visible spectrophotometer [6, 20]. From above evaluation tests, optimised formulation was confirmed (SD4 in **Table 6**) which was then subjected to *in vitro* dissolution studies.

4.3.5 In vitro *dissolution studies*

In vitro dissolution studies of prepared SDs were carried out in 900 ml of 0.1 N HCl as a medium using USP type 2 test apparatus with three replicates. The paddle rotation speed was 75 rpm and a temperature of 37°C ± 0.5 was maintained. In all experiments, 5 ml of dissolution sample was withdrawn at 5 min interval, filtered using a 0.45-mm Whatman filter, and replaced with an equal volume of fresh medium to maintain a constant total volume. Samples were analysed on UV/Visible spectrophotometer at 276 nm.

4.4 Results and discussions

IR study was carried out to check the compatibility between the selected Polymers, with the drug. When the spectra were compared it was found that there was no shifting of functional peaks and no overlapping of characteristic peaks and also there was no appearance of new peaks. **Figure 5** shows the IR spectra of various samples. No significant change in the IR spectra of diclofenac sodium complexes was obtained, except for the broadening of the peaks. The broadening of peaks may be probably due to the restriction of bending and stretching vibrations of the

Formulation code	Saturation solubility in 0.1 N HCl (mg/ml)	pH dependent solubility in 0.1 N HCl (mg/ml)	Percent drug content (in 50 mg)
Pure DS	0.3886 ± 0.0044	6.020 ± 0.038	—
PM1 (1:1)	0.4481 ± 0.0045	8.328 ± 0.069	82.75 ± 1.54
PM2 (1:2)	0.4603 ± 0.0073	9.765 ± 0.0073	86.68 ± 1.27
PM3 (1:3)	0.5168 ± 0.0034	10.278 ± 0.086	88.01 ± 0.94
PM4 (1:4)	**0.5947 ± 0.0046**	**11.265 ± 0.101**	**90.92 ± 1.44**
SD1 (1:1)	1.1802 ± 0.0136	11.984 ± 0.064	93.87 ± 1.89
SD2 (1:2)	1.2612 ± 0.0097	12.735 ± 0.028	94.50 ± 2.11
SD3 (1:3)	1.4894 ± 0.0036	13.324 ± 0.071	95.16 ± 1.34
SD4 (1:4)	**1.9261 ± 0.0154**	**14.291 ± 0.144**	**96.72 ± 1.53**

Table 6.
Saturation solubility, pH dependent solubility and percent drug content studies of pure DS, SDs and PMs.

molecule. Various SDs of DS were prepared using PEG-6000, as carriers by thermal method (Simple fusion) technique to increase the solubility as well as dissolution of poorly aqueous soluble drug DS. The prepared SDs and PMs of DS were evaluated for saturation solubility, pH dependent solubility; percent drug content and *in vitro* dissolution studies. The saturation solubility and pH dependent solubility of pure DS, various prepared SDs and PMs of DS in 0.1 N HCl were measured and the results are given in **Table 6**. All PMs showed higher saturation solubility as compared with pure DS. Again, SDs of DS showed higher saturation solubility than their respective PMs of DS and carrier. This might be attributable to an improvement of wetting of drug particles and localised solubilisation by the hydrophilic polymeric carriers.

Based on the saturation solubility, pH dependent solubility in 0.1 N HCl and drug content among the 8 formulations, PM4 and SD4 were selected to carry out *in vitro* dissolution study and were compared with that of pure DS. The *in vitro* dissolution study of the pure DS, SD4 and PM4 using PEG-6000 as carrier was carried out in 0.1 N HCl at 37°C ± 1°C for 60 min and it was examined by plotting % drug dissolved against a function of time (**Figure 6**). SD4 and PM4 showed improved dissolution of DS over that of pure DS. Pure DS alone yields the slowest dissolution with only 35.65% drug and the dissolution of PM4 (70.76%) was found to be significantly faster when compared with pure DS. SD4 showed the fastest dissolution (92.99%) than PM4 and pure DS. This observation (**Table 7**) indicated that the increased dissolution of DS from SD4 due to presence of drug in amorphous state as compared PM4 and pure DS. As the proportion of PEG-6000 increased, dissolution rates have also been increased. The improvement of dissolution may be due to its hydrophilic nature of the carrier. Thus it can be concluded that the solubility of the poorly soluble drug, DS can be improved markedly by using solid dispersion technique and the carrier, PEG-6000 has increased the dissolution of the drug.

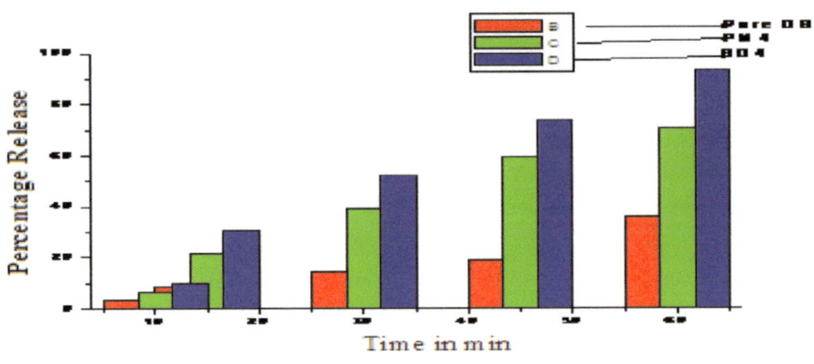

Figure 6.
Dissolution of the pure DS, SD4 and PM4.

	Percentage of diclofenac sodium dissolved from				
***Time in min*/formulation code**	**10**	**15**	**30**	**45**	**60**
Pure DS	3.37	8.50	14.35	18.85	35.65
PM4	6.67	21.23	39.44	59.41	70.76
SD4	**9.73**	**30.51**	**52.25**	**74.00**	**92.99**

Table 7.
Dissolution of the pure DS, SD4 and PM4.

4.5 Preparation of floating gastro retentive tablets

Various ratios of solid dispersions of diclofenac sodium with PEG-6000 were evaluated for percent drug content and out of them the best ratio was selected for preparation of floating tablet of diclofenac sodium. Tablets were prepared by conventional wet granulation method using HPMC K4M, HPMC K15M as a release retardant, carbopol as a swelling agents and $NaHCO_3$ as gas generating agent. Citric acid was also incorporated in the formulation to provide sufficiently acidic medium for $NaHCO_3$ to react and maintain buoyancy. The composition of various formulations is given in **Table 8**. All ingredients (except gas generating agents and magnesium stearate) were passed through sieve no. 60 and mixed in a polybag for 10 min and granulated using PVP K30 (in isopropyl alcohol). The wet mass was passed through sieve number 14 and dried in hot air oven at 50°C for 1.5 h. Dried granules were mixed with magnesium stearate as lubricant, talc as glidant and compressed using 16-station rotary tablet press (Rimek Minipress-I, India) using 13 mm flat punch in order to obtain controlled release floating gastro retentive tablets containing 50 mg of diclofenac sodium. Prior to compression, granules were evaluated for their flow and compressibility characteristic.

4.6 Characterisation of granules

4.6.1 Drug-polymer interaction studies

To study the interaction between drug and polymer, interaction study were performed, drug polymer study were carried out according to the following procedure. Drug and polymer were mixed in 1:1 ratio and put into the glass vials. The glass vials were sealed and placed in the stability chamber at 40°C and 75% RH for 21 days. The sample was analysed for colour change, liquification and bad odours after 7, 15 and 21 days. The IR spectra were taken after 21 days and analysed for any shift in major peaks. No shift was observed in the IR spectrum and no additional peak observed indicating no interaction between drug and polymer.

Ingredient (mg)	Formulation code					
	F1	F2	F3	F4	F5	F6
SD4 (solid dispersion of diclofenac sodium)	250	250	250	250	250	250
HPMC K4	70	—	93	—	105	—
HPMC K15M	—	70	—	93	—	105
Carbopol 934P	70	70	47	47	105	105
Sodium bicarbonate	45	45	45	45	65	65
Citric acid	30	30	30	30	40	40
Avicel PH 102	50	50	50	50	50	50
Magnesium stearate	5	5	5	5	5	5
PVP K-30 5% PVP IN IPA						
Total weight	520	520	520	520	620	620

Table 8.
Composition of different formulations of diclofenac sodium floating tablets.

4.6.2 I-R spectrum of pure drug

About 1 mg of the sample and 100 mg of the potassium bromide (KBr) was taken in a mortar and triturated. A small amount of triturated sample was taken into a pellet maker and compressed at 10 kg/cm$^{2.}$ The pellet was kept onto the sample holder and scanned from 4000 to 400 cm^{-1}.The I-R spectrum of drug sample was obtained using FTIR-8400 s, Shimadzu (**Figure 2**).

4.6.3 I-R spectra for diclofenac sodium with HPMC K4M + HPMC K15M and carbopol 934P

Sample mixture of diclofenac sodium with HPMC K4M + HPMC K15M and carbopol 934P were prepared in KBr discs (1 mg sample in 100 mg KBr). A small amount of triturated sample was taken into a pellet maker and was compressed at 10 kg/cm^2. The scanning range was 4000–400 cm^{-1}, and the resolution was 4 cm^{-1} (**Figures** 7 and **8**).

4.7 Evaluation of granules properties

4.7.1 Angle of repose

The angle of repose of was determined by the funnel method. The accurately weighed granules were taken in a funnel. The height of the funnel was adjusted in such a way that the tip of the funnel just touched the apex of the heap of the granules. The granules were allowed to flow through the funnel freely onto the surface [9, 21]. The diameter of the powder cone was measured and angle of repose was calculated using the following equation.

$$\theta = \tan^{-1}(h/r) \qquad (2)$$

where, h and r are the height and radius of the powder pile, respectively.

4.7.2 Bulk density

Both bulk density (BD) and tapped bulk density (TBD) were determined. A quantity of 2 g of powder from each formula, previously lightly shaken to break any

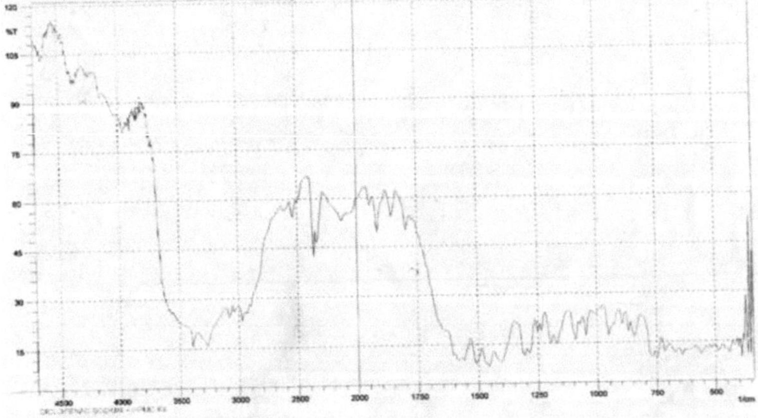

Figure 7.
FTIR of diclofenac sodium + HPMC K4M + HPMC K15M.

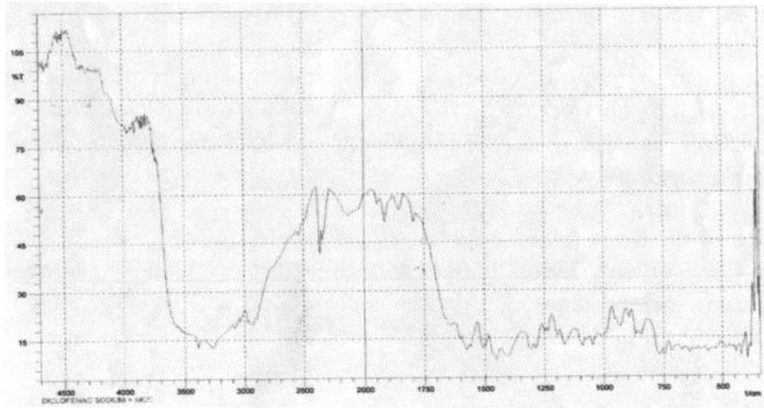

Figure 8.
FTIR of diclofenac sodium + carbopol 934P.

agglomerates formed, was introduced into a 10 ml measuring cylinder [9]. After the initial volume was observed, the cylinder was allowed to fall under its own weight on to a hard surface from the height of 2.5 cm at 2 s intervals. The tapping was continued until no further change in volume was noted.

BD and TBD were calculated using the following formulas.

$$\text{BD} = \text{Weight of the Powder/Volume of the packing.} \tag{3}$$

$$\text{TBD} = \text{Weight of the powder/Tapped volume of the packing.} \tag{4}$$

4.7.3 Compressibility index/carr's index

The flow property was also determined by measuring the compressibility index. It is an important measure that can be obtained from the BD and TBD. According to the theory, the less compressible materials are more flowable. A material having values of less than 20–30% is defined as the free flowing material [9, 21]. Based on the BD and TBD, the percentage compressibility of the bulk drug was determined by using the following formula.

$$\text{Compressibility Index} = \frac{\text{Tap density–Bulk density}}{\text{Tap density}} \times 100 \tag{5}$$

4.8 Evaluation of floating tablets

4.8.1 In vitro *buoyancy determination studies*

In vitro buoyancy studies were performed for all the formulations as per the method described by Rosa *et al* [22]. The randomly selected tablets from each formulation were kept in a 100 ml beaker containing simulated gastric fluid, pH 1.2 as per USP. The time taken for the tablet to rise to the surface and float was taken as floating lag time (FLT). The duration of time the dosage form constantly remained on the surface of medium was determined as the total floating time (TFT) [9, 23–25].

4.8.2 General characteristic

The formulated tablets were assessed for its general appearance.

4.8.2.1 Thickness and diameter

Thickness and diameter of tablets was determined using vernier calliper. Three tablets from each batch were used, and average values were calculated.

4.8.2.2 Weight variation

Formulated floating tablets were tested for weight uniformity, 20 tablets were weighed collectively and individually. From the collective weight, average weight was calculated. Each tablet weight was then compared with average weight to ascertain whether it is within permissible limits or not.

4.8.2.3 Friability test

The Roche friability test apparatus was used to determine the friability of the tablets. 20 pre-weighed tablets were placed in the apparatus, which was given 100 revolutions, after which the tablets were reweighed. The percentage friability was calculated.

$$\%F = \{1 - (\text{loss in weight}/\text{initial weight})\} \times 100 \quad (6)$$

4.8.2.4 Hardness test

Hardness of the tablet was determined using the monsanto hardness tester. The lower plunger was placed in contact with the tablet and a zero reading was taken. The plunger was then forced against a spring by tuning a threaded bolt until the tablet fractured. As the spring was compressed a pointer rides along a gauge in the barrel to indicate the force.

4.8.2.5 Percent drug content

Ten tablets were weighed and powdered. An amount of the powder equivalent to 50 mg of diclofenac sodium was dissolved in 100 ml of 0.1 N HCl, filtered, diluted suitably and analysed for drug content at 276 nm using UV/Visible spectrophotometer.

4.8.2.6 Determination of percent swelling index (percentage water uptake)

The swelling properties of floating tablet containing drug were determined by placing the tablet matrices in the dissolution test apparatus, in 900 ml of distilled water at 37°C ± 0.5°C paddle rotated at 50 rpm. The tablets were removed periodically from dissolution medium. After draining free from water by blotting paper, these were measured for weight gain. Swelling characteristics were expressed in terms of percentage water uptake (%WU) according to the equation shows relationship between swelling index and time.

$$WU\% = \frac{\text{Weight of swollen tablet–Initial weight of the tablet}}{\text{Initial weight of the tablet}} \times 100 \quad (7)$$

4.8.2.7 Dissolution studies using USP type II apparatus with wire sinker

Dissolution test was carried out using USP type II apparatus with wire sinker. The drug release study was carried out for 12 hr. in 900 ml of 0.1 N HCl dissolution media, maintained at 37°C ± 0.5°C and agitated at 50 rpm. Periodically 5 ml samples were withdrawn and filtered through whatman filter paper and samples were replaced by its equivalent volume of dissolution media. The absorbance of DS was measured UV/Visible spectrophotometrically at 276 nm. The percentage cumulative drug release was calculated and amount of CP released from tablets was determined. The floating tablet is wound with the helical wire sinker.

4.8.2.8 Kinetic of drug release

The result of *in vitro* dissolution studies of tablet were fitted with various kinetics models, like zero order (% cumulative drug release vs. time), first order (log % drug remaining vs. time), Higuchi's model (% cumulative drug release vs. square root of time) but these models failed to explain drug release mechanism due to swelling (upon hydration) along with gradual erosion of the matrix. Therefore the dissolution data were also fitted to well-known Korsmeyer and Peppas semi-empirical model to ascertain the mechanism of drug release.

$$\mathbf{log}\ (Mt/M\infty) = \log k + n \log t \tag{8}$$

Where, M∞ is the amount of drug release after infinite time; k is the release rate constant which considers structural and geometric characteristics of the tablets; and n is the diffusional exponent; indicative of the mechanism of drug release. **Table 9** shows an analysis of diffusional release mechanism obtained by various value of n. The criteria for selecting the most appropriate model were chosen on the basis of goodness of fit test. The data were processed for regression analysis using MS EXCEL statistical function.

4.8.2.9 Biodegradability studies of floating tablet

The biodegradability studies were carried out using USP rotating basket apparatus. A tablet (50 mg) were introduced into the baskets which were rotated at 50 rpm in 900 ml of different pH buffer solution (5.0, 6.8, 8.0) maintained at 37°C ± 0.5°C.

4.8.2.10 Stability studies

To assess the drug and formulation stability, stability studies were done according to ICH guidelines. The promising formulation F4 was tested for accelerated testing for a period of 2 months at 40°C ± 2°C/ 75% RH ±5% for their drug content and other parameters.

S. No	n value	Mechanism
1	$n \leq 0.5$	Quasi-fickian diffusion
2	0.5	Fickian diffusion
3	$0.5 \geq n \leq 1.0$	Anomalous (non-fickian) diffusion
4	$n \geq 1.0$	Non-fickian super case 11
5	1	Non-fickian case 11

Table 9.
Release mechanism with variation of n values.

5. Result and discussion

The effervescent floating tablets of SDs of DS were formulated in 6 different batches F1 to F6 by using hydrophilic polymers HPMC K4M, HPMC K15M and hydrophobic polymer carbopol 934P along with effervescing agents, sodium bicarbonate and citric acid (**Table 8**). All the formulations were prepared by wet granulation method. In order to get the longer duration of floating time the high viscosity polymer selected, HPMC K4M was chosen and it was found that, increased viscosity of a polymer prolongs the drug delivery from the dosage form. IR study was carried out to check the compatibility between the selected polymers with the diclofenac sodium drug. This study was performed to assure that there is complete physical entrapment of the drug into the polymer matrix without any mutual interaction. IR spectra were taken for samples like pure drug, and drug-polymer physical mixture at a wavelength of between 4000 and 400 cm^{-1}. All the spectra were compared for shifting of major functional peaks and also for the loss of functional peaks for identification of incompatibility, if any. When the spectra were compared it was found that there was no shifting of functional peaks and no overlapping of characteristic peaks and also there was no appearance of new peaks. **Figures 2**, **7** and **8** shows the IR spectra of various samples. No significant change in the IR spectra of diclofenac sodium complexes was obtained, except for the broadening of the peaks. The broadening of peaks may be probably due to the restriction of bending and stretching vibrations of the molecule [6]. The preformulation studies such as angle of repose, bulk density, tapped density, and carr's index evaluated were found to be within prescribed limits and indicated good free flowing property (**Table 10**).

In vitro Buoyancy of all the prepared tablets formulations were determined using 100 ml beaker containing 0.1NHCl medium shown in (**Table 11**) and the results can be concluded that the batch F3 containing HPMCK4M and carbopol 934P in higher concentration showed good buoyancy lag time is 4.3 min and total floating time is 15 hrs. TFT depends upon the amount of HPMC as the polymer content increased the floating time was increased due to the formation of thick gel which entrapped the gas formed due to $NaHCO_3$ firmly. Among these formulations, the *in vitro* buoyancy was increased in the following order: F3 > F1 > F4 > F2 > F5 > F6. The **Table 9** revealed that FLT minimum for F3 formulation, while its TFT was maximum i.e. 24 h; hence, F3 was selected for further evaluations and *in vitro* drug dissolution studies.

Formulation F3 was evaluated for physical characters like tablet thickness, diameter, hardness, friability, weight variation, percent swelling index, *in vitro* drug release studies. The thickness, diameter and hardness of the formulations satisfied the acceptance criteria. The friability and weight variation was found to be within the limits specified in pharmacopoeia. The drug content was found

Parameter	F1	F2	F3	F4	F5	F6
Angle of repose	22.53°	22.17°	23.42°	21.57°	22.87°	23.34°
Bulk density	0.953 ± 0.026	0.948 ± 0.031	0.975 ± 0.0.098	0.881 ± 0.102	0.836 ± 0.057	0.899 ± 0.083
Tapped density	1.05 ± 0.011	1.041 ± 0.019	1.031 ± 0.026	0.978 ± 0.020	0.981 ± 0.017	0.969 ± 0.038
Carr's index	7.64 ± 0.94	6.66 ± 0.71	5.69 ± 0.56	8.99 ± 0.62	8.68 ± 0.83	7.97 ± 0.49

Table 10.
Pre-compression parameters of granules.

Parameter	F1	F2	F3	F4	F5	F6
Floating lag time (FLT) (s)	160	182	158	163	221	223
Total Floating time (TFT) (h)	22	21	24	20	24	21

Table 11.
In vitro *buoyancy determination.*

spectrophotometrically indicating good content uniformity in the prepared formulation results were shown in **Table 12**.

The swelling index was calculated with respect to time. As time increase, the swelling index was increased because weight gain by tablet was increased proportionally with rate of hydration. The direct relationship was observed in **Table 13**.

The floating formulation F3 was subjected for the dissolution studies using USP type II apparatus with wire sinker in 900 ml of 0.1 N HCl medium. The results are given in **Table 14**. The formulation showed a constant rate of release in a sustained manner similar to zero order kinetics with good buoyancy property. Diclofenac sodium effervescent floating controlled release tablet formulation using solid dispersion (F3) showed far better release than marketed products.

5.1 Effect of sodium bicarbonate concentration on lag time of tablets

The concentration of sodium bicarbonate was found to be critical factor that influenced buoyancy of tablets (**Table 15**). Sodium bicarbonate released CO_2 gas that was trapped into the polymeric matrix of HPMC that made the tablets float. Various concentrations of sodium bicarbonate ranging from 5–12% of tablet weight were used. From the results, it was concluded that with the increasing

Formulation code	Thickness (mm)	Hardness (kg/cm^2)	Friability (%)	Weight variation (mg)	Drug content (%)
F1	4.3 ± 0.016	4.8 ± 0.4	0.24 ± 0.08	542.4 ± 1.9	99.86 ± 0.15
F2	4.4 ± 0.013	5.1 ± 0.3	0.51 ± 0.03	555.8 ± 1.5	99.45 ± 0.08
F3	**4.5 ± 0.015**	**5.4 ± 0.6**	0.17 ± **0.04**	**554.3 ± 1.1**	**100.01 ± 0.04**
F4	4.5 ± 0.013	4.9 ± 0.4	0.46 ± 0.03	545.1 ± 1.8	99.96 ± 0.18
F5	5.5 ± 0.014	4.4 ± 0.1	0.35 ± 0.05	649.1 ± 1.7	98.90 ± 1.05
F6	5.7 ± 0.011	5.8 ± 0.3	0.41 ± 0.04	647.3 ± 0.4	99.02 ± 0.01

Table 12.
General characteristic of floating tablets.

% Swelling index (percentage water uptake)	
Time (h)	**Formulation F3**
1	24
2	37
3	48
4	63
5	71
6	88

Table 13.
% Swelling index (percentage water uptake) of floating tablets.

Time (mins)	Marketed tablet (Voveran-50) (% drug release)	Physical mixture	Diclofenac sodium-solid dispersion (% drug release)	Marketed tablet (Voveran-SR100) (%drug release)	Floating tablet of diclofenac sodium solid dispersion (3) (%drug release)
0	0	0.00	0.00	0.000	0.000
15	15.25 ± 0.64	21.23 ± 0.61	30.51 ± 0.54	12.706 ± 0.67	15.266 ± 0.41
30	37.37 ± 0.53	39.44 ± 0.64	52.25 ± 0.49	16.258 ± 1.27	18.365 ± 0.38
60	51.77 ± 0.86	70.76 ± 0.58	92.99 ± 0.78	19.353 ± 0.98	26.548 ± 0.51
90				24.930 ± 0.79	27.897 ± 0.50
120				27.966 ± 0.93	31.377 ± 0.43
150				32.220 ± 0.76	38.323 ± 0.45
180				38.922 ± 1.22	45.233 ± 0.29
210				45.875 ± 0.96	54.320 ± 0.27
240				51.519 ± 1.23	61.522 ± 0.30
270				60.865 ± 1.31	64.267 ± 0.31
300				64.037 ± .55	69.613 ± 0.35
330				68.561 ± 1.53	73.670 ± 0.51
360				73.686 ± 0.77	76.568 ± 0.42
390				77.371 ± 1.16	80.179 ± 0.44
420				82.957 ± 0.98	85.363 ± 0.47
450				86.414 ± 0.74	87.573 ± 0.58
480				89.213 ± 1.78	96.769 ± 1.19

Table 14.
Comparative in vitro *release study of marketed tablets, physical mixture, solid dispersion and floating tablets of diclofenac solid dispersion.*

S. No.	Concentration of sodium bicarbonate (%)	Floating lag time (s)
1	5	280
2	6	220
3	7	198
4	8	164
5	9	158
6	10	159
7	11	160
8	12	165

Table 15.
Comparison of floating lag time prepared from concentration of sodium bicarbonate.

concentration of sodium bicarbonate, the lag time decreased. A concentration of 8.5–9% w/w sodium bicarbonate was found to be optimal that resulted in tablets having lag time < 3 min and floating time of over 12 h. Similar conclusions were also drawn by other researchers working on floating delivery systems. In both the reported works, optimum concentration of sodium bicarbonate was found to be around 10% w/w of the tablet weight [26, 27] which is slightly higher than our optimal concentration.

5.2 Effect of HPMC grade on lag time of tablets

It was interesting to note that the grade and quantity of HPMC used in the formulations has impact on floating lag time of the tablet. With the increasing molecular weight/quantity of HPMC, the viscosities of the gel matrix around the tablet also increased which in turn in- creased the floating lag time. The lag time for HPMC K15M tablets was slightly higher compared to HPMC K4M tablet. This may be attributed to the increased density of tablet with increasing molecular weight of HPMC (**Table 16**).

5.3 Kinetic of drug release

The various release kinetic models (**Figures 9–12**) were applied to determine the mechanism of drug release from gastro retentive floating tablets and the data is tabulated in **Table 17**. The *in vitro* drug release of optimised formulation (F3) showed the highest regression coefficient values for zero order model, thus indicating absolute correlation between the two variables for the zero order model. Optimised formulations followed Zero order equation proving that the release is by diffusion mechanism. The values of release exponent (n) were calculated from korsmeyer and peppas equation and the 'n' value was determined to be 0.5665 indicating **Anomalous (non-fickian) diffusion.**

So it can be conclude that the optimised formulation follows the zero order plot to a major extend along with other plots to some extent.

S. No.	Quantity of HPMC (mg)	Floating lag time (s)
1	70 (HPMC K4M)	160
2	93 (HPMC K4M)	158
3	105 (HPMC K4M)	163
4	70 (HPMC K15M)	182
5	93 (HPMC K15M)	221
6	105 (HPMC K15M)	223

Table 16.
Comparison of floating lag time prepared from different grade or quantity of HPMC.

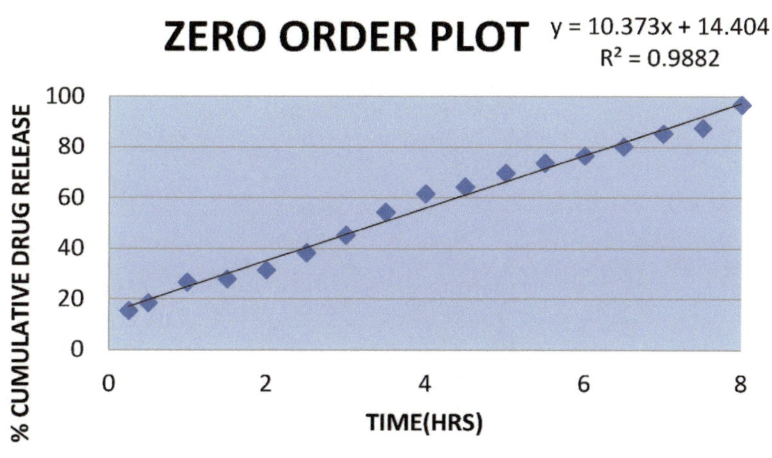

Figure 9.
Zero order release kinetics of optimised formulation.

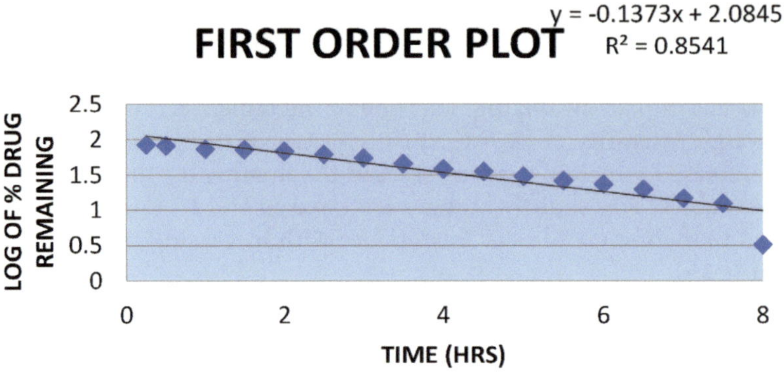

Figure 10.
First order release kinetics of optimised formulation.

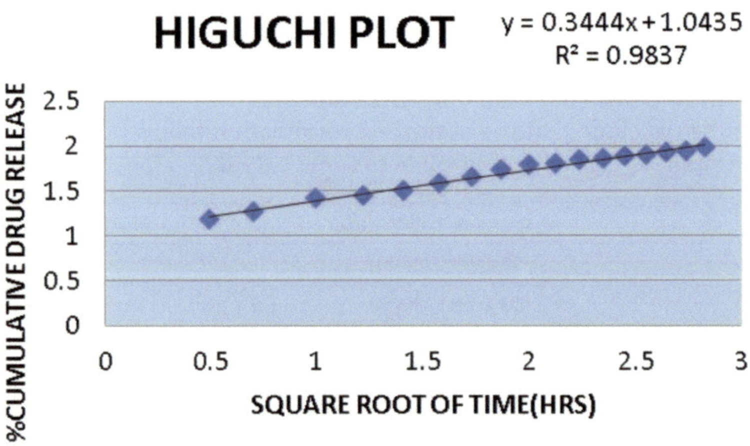

Figure 11.
Higuchi kinetics of optimised formulation.

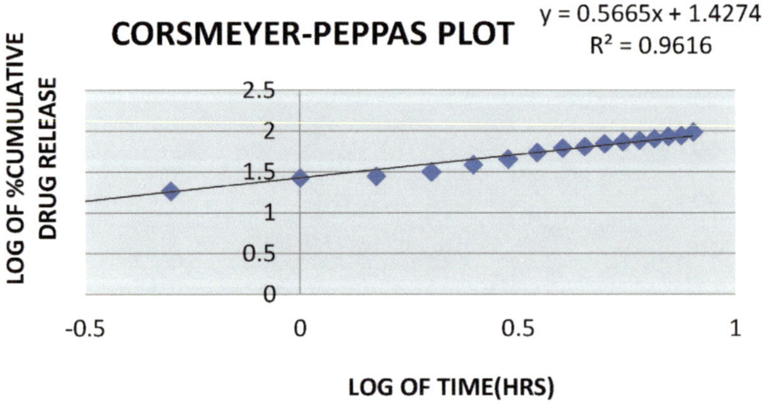

Figure 12.
Korsmeyer-Peppas kinetics of optimised formulation.

S.No	Formulation	Zero order		First order		Higuchi		Korsmeyer-peppas	
1	F3	K	R^2	K	R^2	K	R^2	N	R^2
		10.373	0.9882	−0.1373	0.8541	0.3444	0.9837	0.5665	0.9616

Table 17.
Release kinetic equation values of the optimised formulations.

5.4 Biodegradability studies of floating tablet

Biodegradability studies revealed that the gastro retentive floating tablet of diclofenac (F3) was found to disintegrate and dissolve in intestinal pH within 3 h (**Figure 13**).

Formulation F3 seemed to completely biodegrade in intestinal fluid, and it is the pH of media, which is responsible for slow dissolution of the tablet in intestinal fluid. This indicates that after gastric emptying the regular shaped tablet, gradually become rough with an irregular surface and thereafter was degraded. Thus the gastro retentive floating tablets of diclofenac proved to be suitable gastro retentive dosage form, as they have a rigid structure that resist biodegradation in gastric pH but exhibit complete biodegradation in phosphate buffer pH 8.0.

5.5 Stability studies

Pharmaceutical dosage forms are complex systems composed not only of drug substances but also of various excipients. These excipients, which are non-therapeutic, are intended to contribute desirable, practical properties to the dosage form. These dosage forms may undergo both chemical and physical degradation [28]. Thus, the success of the effective formulation can be evaluated only through the stability studies. This study pursues two particular aims:

- Determination of the optimum formulation and shelf life during developmental stages.

- Derivation of the stability of a product, which guarantees the safety and efficacy of the product up to end of the shelf life at a defined storage condition and pack profile.

So, stability of a pharmaceutical product may be defined as the capability of a particular formulation in a specific container, to remain in its physical, chemical, microbiological, therapeutic and toxicological specifications. Ability of a

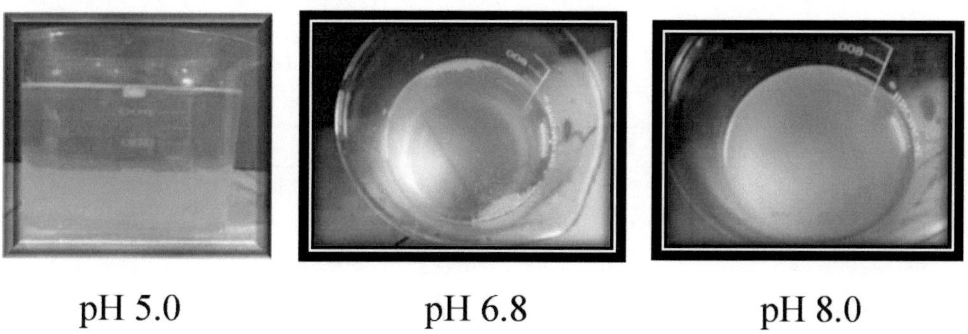

Figure 13.
Images of complete biodegradation of F3 floating tablet after 3 h.

formulation to retain properties in specified limits throughout its shelf-life is referred as stability [28].

The stability of finished pharmaceutical products depends on several factors. On the one hand, it depends on environmental factors such as ambient temperature, humidity and light. On the other hand, it depends on product related factors such as chemical and physical properties of active substance and pharmaceutical excipients, the dosage form and its composition, the manufacturing process, the nature of container closure system and properties of packaging materials.

A study of stability of a pharmaceutical product is essential for safety of the patients, legal requirements concerned with the identity, strength, purity and quality of the drug and to prevent the economic repercussions of marketing an unsuitable product [29, 30].

5.5.1 Experimental

Optimised formulations were stored in screw capped small glass bottles at room temperature and in stability chamber at 40 ± 1°C and 75% relative humidity. Samples were analysed for physical appearance, Hardness (kg/cm^2), Friability (%), Uniformity of weight (mg), Drug content (%), Thickness (mm), Buoyancy lag time (s), Floating time (h) and *in vitro* release after a period of 15, 30, 45, 60, 75, 90 days. Initial drug content was taken as 100% for each formulation. Observations are recorded in **Tables 18** and **19**.

5.5.1.1 Physical characteristics

Various physical parameters were evaluated such as appearance, Buoyancy lag time (s), floating time. Observations are recorded in **Table 18**.

S. No.	Physical parameters	0 days	15th days	30th days	60th days	90th days
1	Appearance	+	+	+	+	+
2	Floating time	+	+	+	+	+
3	Buoyancy lag time (s)	+	+	+	+	+

+, *no change.*

Table 18.
Effect of ageing on physical parameters.

Parameter	Optimised formulation (F3) (n = 3)			
	At 0 day	At 15 days	At 30 days	At 60 days
Hardness (kg/cm^2)	5.4 ± 0.08	5.4 ± 0.1	5.4 ± 0.09	5.2 ± 0.07
Friability (%)	0.17 ± 0.02	0.17 ± 0.01	0.19 ± 0.02	0.20 ± 0.01
Uniformity of weight (mg)	554.3 ± 1.1	554.3 ± 1.1	554.3 ± 1.1	554.3 ± 1.1
Drug content (%)	100.01 ± 0.04	100.01 ± 0.04	99.50 ± 0.58	98.89 ± 0.12
Thickness (mm)	4.55 ± 0.12	4.55 ± 0.09	4.55 ± 0.10	4.55 ± 0.11

Table 19.
Effect of ageing on physico-chemical parameters of optimised formulation.

5.5.1.2 Physcio-chemical parameters

Various parameters were evaluated such as Hardness (kg/cm^2), Friability (%), Uniformity of weight (mg), Drug content (%), Thickness (mm), and *in vitro* release after a period of 15, 30, 45, 60, 75, 90 days. Observations are recorded in **Table 19**.

5.5.1.3 Drug content was assayed by U.V. spectrophotometry

Gastro retentive floating tablet of diclofenac sodium (50 mg) was dissolved in 100 ml of 0.1 N HCl (pH 1.2) by stirring for 6 h using magnetic stirrer. The resulting solution was then filtered using 0.45 m millipore filter, 1 ml of this solution was taken and added to 100 ml of 0.1 N HCl (pH 1.2). It was then analysed spectrophotometrically at the predetermined λ max (276 nm) to determine concentration of the drug. The determinations were made in triplicate.

5.5.1.4 In vitro *dissolution studies*

In vitro dissolution studies were carried out using simulated gastric fluid (pH 1.2).

5.5.2 Result and discussion

5.5.2.1 Physical parameters of the optimised tablets formulation

The Physical parameters after 15th, 30th, 60th, 90th days are as mentioned in **Table 18**. All the Physical parameter are within the acceptable limits which indicated that gastro retentive floating tablet of diclofenac sodium showed no significant change in the physical appearance at room temperature and in stability chamber at 40°C ± 2°C and 75 ± 5% relative humidity indicating that the formulations were physically stable at these temperatures.

5.5.2.2 Physico-chemical parameters of the optimised formulation

Various parameters were evaluated such as Hardness (kg/cm^2), Friability (%), Uniformity of weight (mg), Drug content (%), Thickness (mm), and *in vitro* release

S. No.	Sampling interval (days)	% Residual drug content Mean ± S.D. (n = 3)	
		At room temp.	At 40 ± 2°C/75 ± 5% RH
1	0	100.01 ± 0.03	100.01 ± 0.03
2	15	99.82 ± 0.12	99.66 ± 0.09
3	30	99.56 ± 0.09	99.25 ± 0.18
4	45	98.75 ± 0.14	98.40 ± 0.15
5	60	98.56 ± 0.05	97.72 ± 0.9
6	75	98.07 ± 0.09	97.51 ± 0.10
7	90	97.69 ± 0.07	96.66 ± 0.06

Table 20.
Effect of ageing on residual drug content at room temperature &40 ± 2 °C/ 75 ± 5%RH.

after a period of 15, 30, 45, 60, 75, 90 days. Observations are recorded in **Table 6**. All the physico-chemical parameters are within the acceptable limits which indicated that formulation were stable over the period of 90 days.

5.5.2.3 Residual drug content of stability batch

Initial drug content of formulations was 100.01 ± 0.04.the drug contents at the end of 15th, 30th, 60th, 90th days were found to be as given in **Table 20**. The drug content was within the permissible limits. The percent residual drug content was determined and the log percent residual content was plotted against time t (**Figures 14–17**), which reflected almost linear relationship.

5.5.2.4 In vitro *dissolution studies*

The dissolution results obtained were as given in the **Table 21**.

The dissolution behaviour of samples withdrawn at different interval was similar and the difference in dissolution pattern of samples kept at two different conditions of storage was negligible.

The log % residual drug content vs. time graph was also plotted in order to evaluate shelf-life and half-life of formulations.

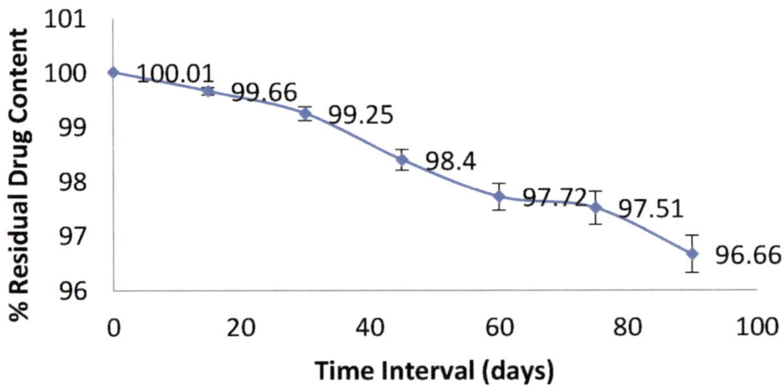

Figure 14.
Effect of ageing on residual drug content at 40 ± 2°C/75 ± 5%RH.

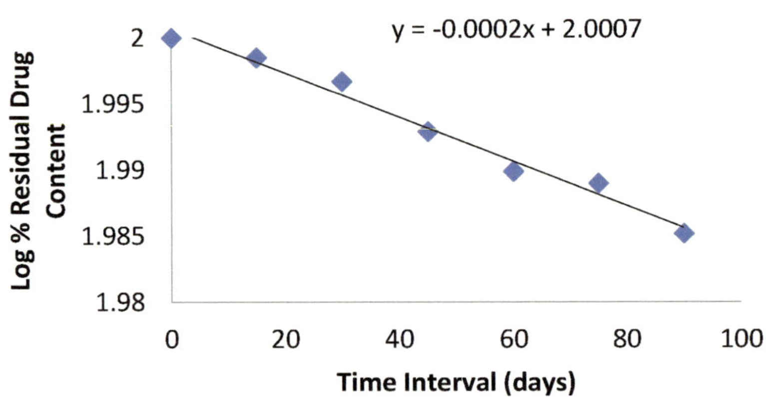

Figure 15.
Plot of log % residual drug content Vs time at 40 ± 2°C/75 ± 5%RH.

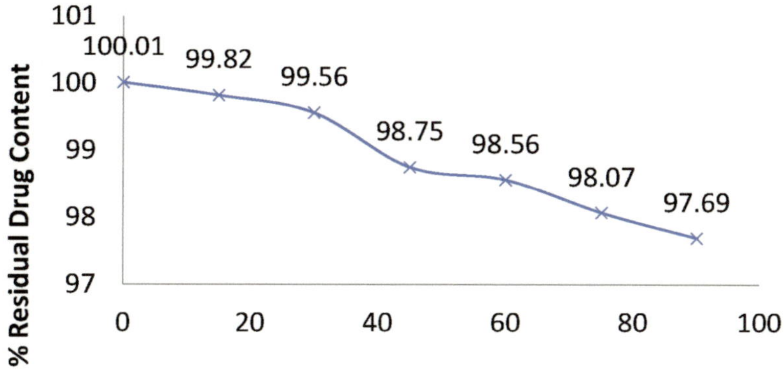

Figure 16.
Effect of ageing on residual drug content at room temperature.

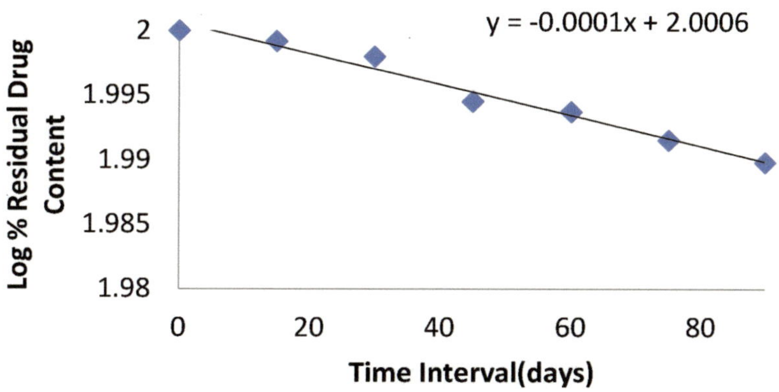

Figure 17.
Plot of log % residual drug content vs. time at room temp.

Time interval (days)	% Cumulative drug release in 8 h ± SD (n = 3)	
	Room temperature	40 ± 2°C/75 ± 5% RH
0	96.769 ± 1.19	96.769 ± 1.19
15	95.78 ± 0.84	94.34 ± 1.52
30	94.81 ± 1.64	93.05 ± 0.81
60	94.45 ± 0.56	92.89 ± 0.69
90	93.97 ± 0.93	92.45 ± 1.21

Table 21.
Effect of ageing on % cumulative drug release at room temperature & 40 ± 2°C/75 ± 5%RH.

Shelf-life was evaluated by the equation:

$$T_{10\%} = 0.104/K \quad (9)$$

Degradation rate constant K was calculated from the slope of straight line between log of % residual drug and time interval. The time required for degradation of 10% drug was calculated as $T_{10\%}$.

S. No.	Storage condition	K (day^{-1})	$T_{10\%}$ (days)	$t_{1/2}$ (days)
1	40 ± 2 °C/75 ± 5%RH	3.822×10^{-4}	272.039	1812.72
2	Room temperature	2.303×10^{-4}	451.58	3009.11

Table 22.
Shelf life of optimised formulation.

Half-life was evaluated by the equation:

$$T_{1/2} = 0.693/K \quad (10)$$

Gastro retentive floating tablet of diclofenac sodium stored at 40 ± 2°C/75 ± 5% RH showed K value as 3.822×10^{-4} and $t_{10\%}$ value as 272.039 days, while those stored at room temperature showed K value as 2.303×10^{-4} and $t_{10\%}$ value as 451.58 days (**Table 22**).

The $T_{10\%}$ obtained in case of formulation stored at 40°C ± 2°C/75 ± 5%RH was found to be lower in comparison with the formulation stored at room temperature which indicated that the formulations tend to degrade faster at higher temperatures and humidity.

The results of stability studies suggest that for adequate shelf life of optimised gastro retentive floating tablet of diclofenac sodium, it should be stored in cool and dry place.

6. Conclusions

In the above research work, ECRFT has been developed by using dual approach; one is solid dispersion (for solubility enhancement) and other is effervescent floating technique (for achieving extended retention in upper G.I.T.), which was prepared from previously optimised solid dispersion of diclofenac sodium. Formulated tablets showed outstanding physicochemical properties, biodegradation studies, stabilities studies, and prolong gastric retention with control release. When compared with marketed tablets of immediate release (Voveran-50) and control release (Voveran-100SR), the optimised formulation F3 was found to be favourable for improving bioavailability of drug, enhancing its therapeutics efficacy and improving patient compliance due to less frequent dosing requirement. Hence, it can be concluded that the prepared formulation can be used positively as a particular oral controlled release-floating tablet for once a day administration.

Acknowledgements

The authors would like to express their hearty gratitude to Kwality Pharmaceutical Pvt Ltd, Amritsar for supplying diclofenac sodium raw material and excipients. We are also thankful to Dr. Abhishek Bansal, Department of Pharmaceutical sciences, Gurukul Kangri University, Haridwar for the help provided during research.

Conflict of interest

There is no conflict of interest.

Acronyms and abbreviations

SEM	scanning electron microscopy
PM	physical mixtures
DT	disintegration time
ECRFT	effervescent controlled release floating tablet
SDs	solid dispersions
DS	diclofenac sodium
BD	bulk density
TBD	tapped bulk density
TFT	total floating time
%WU	percentage water uptake
FLT	floating lag time

Author details

Peeush Singhal[1*], Rajneesh Dutt Kaushik[1] and Vijay Jyoti Kumar[2]

1 Department of Pharmaceutical Sciences (FMSH), Gurukul Kangri Vishwavidyalaya, Haridwar, India

2 Department of Pharmaceutical Sciences, H.N.B. Garhwal Central University, Srinagar, Uttarakhand, India

*Address all correspondence to: peeushpharma@gmail.com

References

[1] Available from: http://www.drugs.com/diclofenac.html

[2] Rao GK, Mandapalli PK, Manthri R, Reddy VP. Development and in vivo evaluation of gastro retentive delivery systems for cefuroxime axetil. Saudi Pharmaceutical Journal. 2013;**21**(1): 53-59. DOI: 10.1016/j.jsps.2012.01.003

[3] Chau Le-Ngoc VO, Chulhun P, Beom-Jin L. Current trends and future perspectives of solid dispersions containing poorly water-soluble drugs review article. European Journal of Pharmaceutics and Biopharmaceutics. 2013;**85**(3) Part B:799-813

[4] Giri TK, Kumar K, Alexander A, Ajazuddin, Badwaik H, Tripathi DK. A novel and alternative approach to controlled release drug delivery system based on solid dispersion technique review article. Bulletin of Faculty Pharmacy, Cairo University. 2012;**50**(2): 147-159

[5] Willis JV, Kendall MJ, Flinn RM, Thornill DP, Welling PG. The pharmacokinetics of diclofenac sodium following intravenous and oral administration. European Journal of Clinical Pharmacology. 1979;**16**(6): 405-410

[6] Sharma N, Jain N, Sudhakar CK, Jain S. Formulation and evaluation of gastro retentive floating tablets containing cefpodoxim proxetil solid dispersions. International Journal of Current Pharmaceutical Research. 2012; **4**(4):82-87

[7] Shivakumar HN, Desai BG, Deshmukh G. Design and optimization of diclofenac sodium controlled release solid dispersions by response surface methodology. Indian Journal of Pharmaceutical Sciences. 2008;**70**(1):22-30

[8] Baumgartner S, Kristl J, Vrecer F, Vodopivec P, Zorko B. Optimization of floating matrix tablets and evaluation of their gastric residence time. International Journal of Pharmaceutics. 2000;**195**:125-135

[9] Chanvanpatil M, Jain P, Chaudhari S, Shear R, Vavia P. Novel sustained release, swellable and bio adhesive gastro retentive drug delivery system for ofloxacin. International Journal of Pharmaceutics. 2006;**316**:86-92

[10] United State Pharmacopoeia 31. The National Formulary. Asian Edition. 26 (I). North Bethesda, Maryland, United States: The Board of Trustees; 2008. pp. 297-298

[11] Seedher N, Bhatia S. Solubility enhancement of cox-2 inhibitors using various solvent systems. AAPS PharmSciTech. 2003;**4**(3):33

[12] Instruction manual pharmaspec. UV-1700 Series. User's System Guide. Kyoto Japan: Shimadzu Corporation;

[13] Pavia LK. Introduction to Spectroscopy. 3rd ed. United States: Thomson Brooks/Cole; 2001. p. 358

[14] ICH Harmonized Tripartite Guideline, Text on Validation of Analytical Procedure (Q2A). London, UK: EMEA; 1994

[15] Beckett AH, Stenlake JB. Practical Pharmaceutical Chemistry. 4th ed. Vol. 2. London, UK; 2007. pp. 282-288

[16] Garatt DC. The Quantitative Analysis of Drugs. 3rd ed. CBS publishers and Distributors; 2005. p. 876

[17] British Pharmacopoeia. The British pharmacopoeia commission offices, London. 2008;**1&2**:685-686

[18] Indian Pharmacopoeia. The Controlled Publication, New Delhi. Vol. 2. 2007. pp. 402-403

[19] Sharma BK. Instrumental Methods of Chemical Analysis. 23rd ed. Goel Publishing House; 2004. pp. 292-302

[20] Barzegar-Jalali M, Alaei-Beirami M, Javadzadeh Y, Mohammadi G, Hamidi A, Andalib S, et al. Comparison of physicochemical characteristics and drug release of diclofenac sodium-eudragit® RS100 nanoparticles and solid dispersions. Powder Technology. 2012;**219**:211-216

[21] Davis SS, Stockwel AF, Taylor MJ, Hardy JG, Whalley DR, Wilson CG. The effect of density on the gastric emptying of single and multiple unit dosage forms. Pharmaceutical Research. 1986;**3**:208-213

[22] Rosa M, Zia H, Rhodes T. Design and testing in vitro of a bioadhesive and floating drug delivery system for oral application. International Journal of Pharmaceutics. 1994;**105**:65-70

[23] Li S, Lin S, Daggy BP, Mirchandani HL, Chien YW. Effect of HPMC and carbopol on the release and floating properties of gastric floating drug delivery system using factorial design. International Journal of Pharmaceutics. 2003;**253**:13-22

[24] Machida Y, Inouy K, Tokumura T, Iwata M, Nagai T. Preparation and evaluation of intragastric buoyant preparations. Drug Design and Delivery. 1989;**4**:155-161

[25] Moes AJ. Gastro retentive dosage forms. Critical Reviews in Therapeutic Drug Carrier Systems. 1993;**10**:143-159

[26] Dhumal RS, Rajmane ST, Dhumal ST, Pawar AP. Design and evaluation of bi-layered floating tablets of cefuroxime axetil for bimodal release. Journal of Scientific and Industrial Research. 2006;**65**:812-816

[27] Patel VF, Patel NM. Intragastricoating drug delivery system of cefuroxime axetil: In vitro evaluation. AAPS PharmSciTech. 2006;**7**:E1-E7

[28] Yoshika S, Stell VJ. Stability of Drugs and Dosage Forms. 2nd ed. New Delhi: Springer Private Ltd; 2006. pp. 151-186

[29] Garret NM. Stability studies of floating drug delivery dosage form. Journal of Pharmaceutical Sciences. 1965;**54**:1557

[30] Gennaro AR. Remington: Pharmaceutical Sciences and Practice of Pharmacy. 20th ed. Vol. 1. Philadelphia: Lippincott Williams & Wilkins; 1990. p. 986

Section 2

Pharmaceutical Dosage Forms

Chapter 3

3D-Printed Modified-Release Tablets: A Review of the Recent Advances

Angeliki Siamidi, Eleni Tsintavi, Dimitrios M. Rekkas and Marilena Vlachou

Abstract

The broad spectrum of applications of three-dimensional printing (3D printing, 3DP) has attracted the attention of researchers working in diverse fields. In pharmaceutics, the main idea behind 3D printing products is to design and develop delivery systems that are suited to an individual's needs. In this way, the size, appearance, shape, and rate of delivery of a wide array of medicines could be easily adjusted. The aim of this chapter is to provide a compilation of the 3D printing techniques, used for the fabrication of oral drug delivery systems, and review the relevant scientific developments in particular those with modified-release characteristics.

Keywords: 3D printing, modified release, oral drug delivery, tablets

1. Introduction

3D printing is an object fabrication technique based on the sequential deposition of layers of materials. Using a computer-aided design (CAD) software, structures of various sizes and shapes can be produced. This method has found application in many sectors, from industrial engineering to personalized biomaterials and devices in medicine [1, 2]. Within the pharmaceutical field, 3D printing can produce small batches of medicinal products, with tailored dosages, shapes, sizes, and release characteristics [3]. These advantages of 3D printing facilitate the efforts towards personalized therapies. The need for the modification of a dose that will fit better a patient's individual needs arises from differences in the patient's age, weight, and severity of disease(s) [4]. Even though there are great advancements in drug administration methods, the orally administered drugs remain the most preferred choice by patients due to the fact that it is relatively safe, very convenient and cost-effective. The preference on oral solid pharmaceutical forms, especially tablets, has rendered the personalization of oral solid dosage forms a step forward in the healthcare system [4].

2. History

The increasing applications of 3D printing have made it a well-accepted concept at present times. Charles Hull is considered the pioneer of 3D printing, as he developed, patented, and commercialized the first equipment for the 3D printing of objects in 1983. Hull's 3D printing technique was based on stereolithography. It consisted of a laser that moved across the surface of a liquid resin, curing it. This process was repeated layer by layer many times until the desired shape was formed. In 1988, Charles Deckard filed a patent for selective laser sintering. In this process, a laser beam is scanned over a powder bed to sinter or fuse the powder that is placed on a powder bed. The powder bed is then lowered, fresh powder is spread, and the process is repeated to produce a solid object. The un-bonded is then removed, and the structure can be further treated, for example, with heat, to enforce the bonding. In 1989, Scott Crump filed a patent on fused deposition modeling. Using this technique, the object is formed by depositing layers of solidifying materials (self-hardening waxes, thermoplastic resins, and molten metals) until the desired shape is formed [5, 6]. In 2015, the FDA approved Spritam®, the first 3D-printed prescription drug product to treat partial onset seizures, myoclonic seizures, and primary generalized tonic-clonic seizures. Since then, many innovations have been evolved using the 3DP technology.

3. Advantages and limitations

The oral dosage form production by the 3DP processes has many advantages specially for customizing drug delivery. The active ingredient can be included in the dosage form as per each patient requirements to achieve a personalized dose and release pattern. 3D printing aids also in achieving multidrug combinations with complex release profiles [7]. On-demand production and tailor-made products with specific geometries, designs, and shape forms can be achieved which otherwise would be difficult with the conventional tableting. Even though there has been intense research to circumvent the 3D printing flaws, this new technology has still some limitations. Few 3D printing techniques may produce relatively porous structures and uneven shapes of dosage forms [6]. When fused deposition modeling technique is utilized, the use of only thermostable drugs and the few available compatible excipients is a limiting step. Also, with stereolithography, the challenge lies on the potential drug degradation due to the exposure to UV light that induces polymerization reaction [5].

4. Various techniques used in 3D printing

Irrespective of the 3D printing technique employed, the process follows three basic steps: the creation of a computer-aided design file; followed by its transformation to a rapid prototyping stereolithography file (.stl), which describes the surface geometry of the 3D object; and finally, its conversion to a machine specific code (.gcode) which is recognized by the 3D printer machine and creates the final object [8] (**Figure 1**).

There are various ways to classify the 3D techniques, according to the additive process followed, the form of the raw materials used, the mechanism of layering, or even the kind of printing heads utilized [9]. **Figure 2** illustrates the different 3D

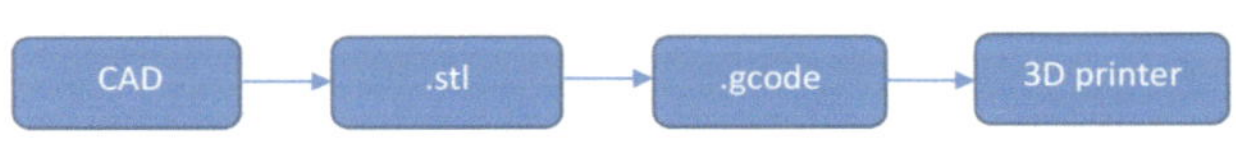

Figure 1.
The basic steps of 3D printing process.

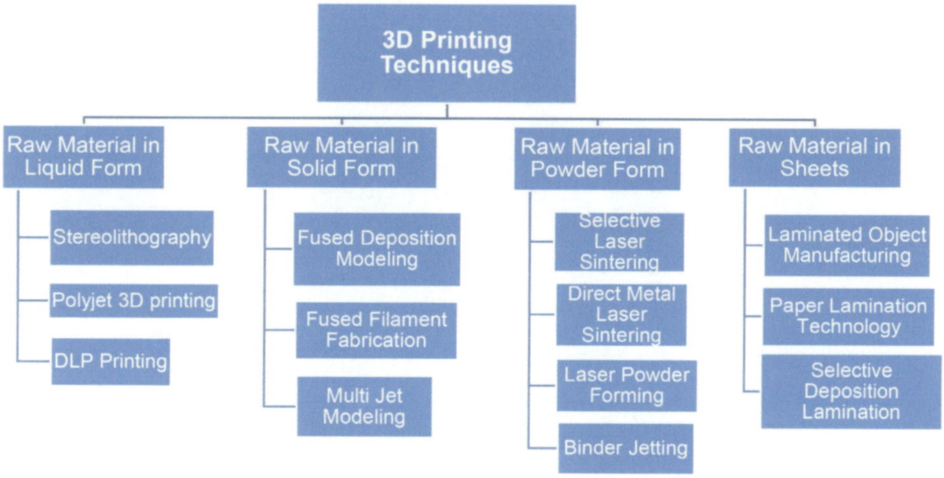

Figure 2.
3D printing technique categorization.

printing techniques categorized by the raw materials employed. Among them, stereolithography, selective laser sintering, binder jetting, and fused deposition modeling are the most used techniques in the literature for the production of pharmaceutical dosage forms [10].

Stereolithography employs raw materials in the liquid form, such as photosensitive/photopolymerizable liquid resins. A high-energy light source like ultraviolet irradiation solidifies the liquid resins, creating the 3D object [6]. Among the advantages of this technique are the high accuracy and good surface quality of the object. This method has been widely used for implant design and manufacture as well as for creating accurate 3D models acquired from various anatomical scans of a patient.

Selective laser sintering (SLS) technique utilizes raw materials in a powder form, and the laser used melts and bonds the layers of material powders together. SLS has been used for the manufacturing of artificial tissue.

On the other hand, binder jetting technique, also called drop-on-demand inkjet printing or 3D printing, is able to create 3D objects from powder materials by depositing liquid binder droplets onto a powder substrate and sticking the particles together [9, 10]. This technique along with the continuous inkjet printing belongs to the printing-based inkjet systems and has been utilized for the fabrication of implants and solid dosage forms, such as the first commercially printed tablet Spritam®.

Finally, the most widely spread technique is the fused deposition modeling (FDM), and it belongs to the nozzle-based printing techniques. FDM is characterized by the use of thermoplastic polymers that pass through a pre-heated printing head and is melted and extruded through a precise nozzle with a specific diameter. In contact with the cold printing surface, the polymers solidify and thus create the 3D object. A variation of this type of 3D printing technique is the semisolid extrusion system, in which semiconductors (gels, ointments) are printed through a syringe-shaped extruder [10]. In the recent years, these techniques have been extensively used for the research and development of various pharmaceutical forms such as hydrogels or coated solid dosage forms [11].

Figure 3 depicts the main additive manufacturing technologies which either experimentally or industrially have been used for the manufacturing of pharmaceutical dosage forms.

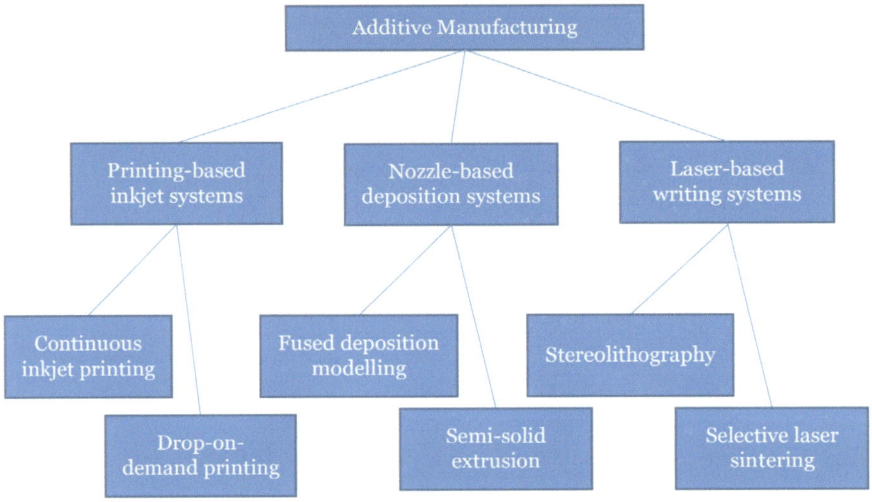

Figure 3.
Basic 3D printing techniques deployed for the manufacturing of pharmaceutical dosage forms.

5. Recent accomplishments in modified-release 3D-printed tablets

Orodispersible, sublingual, fast-dissolving drug delivery formulations that rapidly disintegrate in the oral cavity or immediate-release tablets by 3D printing have been produced [12–15].

Multipurpose therapeutic systems offering tailored combinations of drugs, drug doses, and the desired release kinetic properties have attracted increasing attention, due to the advantages that these personalized pharmaceutical products could offer. In this respect, many scientists have designed modified-release oral dosage medicines, using 3D printing. The drug release from modified-release formulations is changed on purpose from that of an immediate-release formulation to achieve a preferred therapeutic goal. The applications of 3DP on modified *per oral* drug delivery are summarized in **Table 1**.

Genina et al. [16] have shown that coupling fused deposition modeling 3D printing with the hot-melt extrusion offers a new method for manufacturing tailored-dosage medicines, with modified-release properties. In detail an oral dual-compartmental dosage unit (dcDU) has been designed, and the in vitro and in vivo release profiles of an antitubercular drug combination of rifampicin and isoniazid have been evaluated. These two active ingredients are considered as first-line therapy for tuberculosis but interact negatively with each other upon simultaneous release in acidic environment. This was circumvented by the compartmentalization of rifampicin and isoniazid into sealable compartments of 3D-printed dual-compartmental dosage units. This novel delivery system was characterized with focus on microscopic verification of the designed attributes, the modulation of drug release from dcDUs, and the pharmacokinetic profile of dcDUs in rats. In another study [17] an oral solid dosage form was developed by employing the fused deposition modeling, using a custom-built filament consisted of polyvinyl alcohol, mannitol, and hydrochlorothiazide, as a model drug, co-formulated via hot-melt extrusion. The dissolution studies performed demonstrated zero-order release kinetics. In another study [18], hot-melt extrusion and fused deposition modeling were used to produce different shaped tablets (cube, pyramid, cylinder, sphere, and torus) containing acetaminophen. It was found that drug's release was not

Release behavior*	Dosage form	API(s)	Excipient(s)	Technique	Ref.
Modified	Dual-compartment tablet	Rifampicin and isoniazid	Polyethylene oxide, polylactic acid (PLA), polyvinyl alcohol (PVA)	FDM/HME	[16]
	Three-compartment tablet	Hydrochlorothiazide	Partially hydrolyzed PVA (Mowiol®4–88), mannitol	FDM/HME	[17]
	Tablets of various shapes	Paracetamol	Polyvinyl alcohol	FDM/HME	[18]
	Caplets	Budesonide	Polyvinyl alcohol, Eudragit® L 100, triethyl citrate, talc, isopropanol-water solution	FDM/HME and fluid bed coating	[19]
	Tablets	5-Aminosalicylic acid and 4-aminosalicylic acid	Polyvinyl alcohol	FDM	[20]
	Caplets	Paracetamol or caffeine	Polyvinyl alcohol	FDM	[21]
	Tablets	4-Aminosalicylic acid and paracetamol	Polyethylene glycol diacrylate, diphenyl (2,4,6-trimethylbenzoyl) phosphine oxide, and (PEG 300)	Stereolithography	[22]
	Tablets	Acetaminophen	Methocel™ E50, polyvinylpyrrolidone (Povidone K30), ethyl cellulose, Eudragit® RS 100, stearic acid, sodium lauryl sulfate, fluorescein, colloidal silicon dioxide	Inkjet printing	[23]
Extended	Tablets	Acetaminophen	Benecel™ HPMC E5 and Aqualon™ EC N14 with either Klucel™ HPC EF and LF, Soluplus®, or Eudragit® L 100	FDM/HME	[24]
	Tablets	Theophylline	Eudragit RL 100, RS 100, and E and hydroxypropyl cellulose (SSL grade), triethyl citrate	FDM/HME	[25]
	Tablets	Prednisolone	Polyvinyl alcohol	FDM	[26]
	Tablets	Fluorescein	Polyvinyl alcohol	FDM	[27]
Controlled	Tablets	Fenofibrate	White beeswax	Inkjet printing	[28]
Sustained	Polypill	Captopril, nifedipine, and glipizide	Hydroxypropyl methylcellulose (HPMC 2208), polyethylene glycol (PEG 6000),	Extrusion	[29]

Release behavior*	Dosage form	API(s)	Excipient(s)	Technique	Ref.
			tromethamine, lactose, sodium chloride, D-mannitol, croscarmellose sodium, microcrystalline cellulose, sodium starch glycolate, hydroxypropyl methylcellulose (Methocel™), cellulose acetate		
Delayed	DuoCaplet	Paracetamol and caffeine	Polyvinyl alcohol	FDM/HME	[30]
	Tablets	Paracetamol	Hypromellose acetate succinate (HPMC LG, MG, HG), methylparaben NF grade, magnesium stearate	FDM/HME	[31]
	Shell-core tablets	Theophylline, budesonide, and diclofenac sodium	Core: Polyvinylpyrrolidone, triethyl citrate, talc or tribasic phosphate sodium, and API Shell: Eudragit® L 100–55, triethyl citrate, and talc	Dual FDM/HME	[32]
Pulsatile	Two-compartment capsular device	Acetaminophen	Polylactic acid, polyvinyl alcohol, hydroxypropyl methylcellulose (HPMC), HPMC acetate succinate, polyvinyl alcohol-polyethylene glycol graft copolymer, glycerol, polyethylene glycol (PEG 400, PEG8000), blue and yellow dye-containing formulations (Kollicoat®IR Brilliant Blue and Kollicoat®IRyellow)	FDM/HME injection molding	[33]
Immediate /sustained	Bilayer tablet	Guaifenesin	Hydroxypropyl methylcellulose (HPMC 2910 & 2208), poly(acrylic acid), microcrystalline cellulose, sodium starch glycolate	Extrusion	[34]
	Polypill	Aspirin, hydrochlorothiazide, ramipril, pravastatin sodium, atenolol	Cellulose acetate, D-mannitol, polyethylene glycol (PEG 6000) sodium starch glycolate, Polyvinylpyrrolidone	Extrusion	[35]

Release behavior*	Dosage form	API(s)	Excipient(s)	Technique	Ref.
			(Povidon K30), hydroxypropyl methylcellulose (Methocel™ K100MCR), lactose		
Immediate/ extended	Tablets	Chlorpheniramine maleate	Microcrystalline cellulose powder, Eudragit® E 100, RLPO	Inkjet	[36]
Enteric dual pulsatory	Tablets	Diclofenac	Avicel PH301, lactose, Eudragit® L 100,	Inkjet	[36]
Dual pulsatory	Tablets	Diclofenac	Eudragit® E 100 and L 100	Inkjet	[36]

**The release behavior reported as defined by the author.*

Table 1.
An overview of the 3DP technique applications in modified per oral drug delivery (FDM, fused deposition modeling; HME, hot-melt extrusion).

dependent on the tablet surface area, but on the surface-area-to-volume ratio, indicating the effect of the shape on the release profile. The results showed that the tablets of similar mass showed little difference in dissolution profiles that could be explained by the erosion-mediated process that controlled the drug release. Tablets of various shapes may alter the drug dissolution profiles and can aid in the design of new dosage forms with specific pharmacokinetic characteristic targeted to different sites in the gastrointestinal track. Fused deposition 3D printing technology alongside with hot-melt extrusion and fluid bed coating was used to fabricate modified-release budesonide dosage forms. The drug was loaded into polyvinyl alcohol filaments which were then engineered into capsule-shaped tablets and coated with a layer of enteric polymer. The dissolution studies showed that the drug release from the caplet formulation started at the small intestine and continued in a sustained manner throughout the large intestine and colon [19]. The same group of researchers has also produced tablets containing as model drugs the two aminosalicylic acid isomers, 5-aminosalicylic acid and 4-aminosalicylic acid, using fused deposition modeling. The results indicated that the release profiles obtained could be easily modified by the proper selection of the printing parameters [20]. Furthermore, fused deposition modeling was used to produce acetaminophen or caffeine caplets from polyvinyl alcohol filaments. The dissolution tests performed in biorelevant bicarbonate media revealed distinctive modified-release profiles, which were dependent on drug solubility and drug loading. The results indicated that the drug release can be faster from formulations incorporating the drug with higher solubility and higher loading [21]. Additionally, Wang et al. [22] managed to formulate modified-release tablets of paracetamol and 4-aminosalicylic acid using polyethylene glycol diacrylate as monomer and diphenyl (2,4,6-trimethylbenzoyl) phosphine oxide as a photoinitiator in stereolithographic 3D printing. Also, in another study [23], researchers employed the powder bed/jetting method to construct a methacrylic or ethylcellulose matrix tablet to achieve a modified release of acetaminophen. Erosion and in vitro dissolution studies in ethylcellulose-containing tablets indicated that the drug was released via a two-dimensional surface erosion mechanism and 98% of the drug could be released linearly in 12 h. Tablets with other release-retardation materials, such as sodium lauryl sulfate, stearic acid, and

Eudragit RS-100, showed similar release-retardation effects by different release mechanisms.

Zhang et al. fabricated solid-dispersion filaments with acetaminophen dissolved or dispersed in a polymer matrix by hot-melt extrusion technology, which was suitable for fused deposition modeling-based 3D printing. The 3D printed tablets showed more extended drug release rates than the directly compressed tablets [24]. In another study [25], using the same methods, scientists presented a flexible dose tablet system, suitable for both immediate and extended-release tablets. As excipients three methacrylic polymers (Eudragit RL, RS, and E) as well as a cellulose-based material (hydroxypropyl cellulose, HPC SSL) were used, while theophylline was used as a model drug substance. Moreover, in another report [26], the feasibility of using a fused deposition modeling-based 3D printer to fabricate extended-release tablets, using prednisolone loaded poly(vinyl alcohol) filaments, and to control its release was investigated. The results indicated that the in vitro drug release was extended up to 24 h, showing that the fused deposition modeling is a promising method to control the dose of extended-release tablets. Moreover in another work, polyvinyl alcohol filaments have been loaded with fluorescein as a model drug, by swelling of the polymer in ethanolic drug solution, and 10-mm-diameter tablets of polyvinyl alcohol/fluorescein using fused deposition modeling 3DP were printed. The dissolution tests that were conducted in modified Hank's buffer indicated controlled-release profiles [27].

Kyobula et al. [28] have prepared drug-loaded solid dosage forms with complex geometries such as honeycomb based, using hot-melt 3D inkjet printing. The model drug used was fenofibrate, and the relevant studies indicated controlled release. This study verified an alternative production approach for solid dosage forms with different geometry, which could achieve various release profiles for personalized drug products.

Khaled et al. [29] have employed 3D extrusion-based printing as a technique for the production of multi-active tablets with well-defined and separate controlled-release profiles for three different drugs, namely, captopril, nifedipine, and glipizide. This "polypill" incorporated an osmotic pump for captopril and sustained release compartments for nifedipine and glipizide. The dissolution testing showed that the captopril portion exhibited the expected zero-order drug release from an osmotic pump, while the others showed either first-order release or Korsmeyer-Peppas release kinetics dependent on the active/excipient ratio used.

Goyanes et al. [30] used the fused deposition modeling 3D printing to fabricate novel oral drug delivery systems with paracetamol and caffeine filaments of poly (vinyl alcohol), with the intent of applying this process to the production of personalized products, tailored at the point of dispensing or use. The design included a multilayer device, with each layer containing drug, whose identity was different to the drug in the adjacent layers, and a two-compartment device, comprising of a caplet in caplet (DuoCaplet), with each compartment containing a different drug. The drug release tests in biorelevant bicarbonate media showed unique drug release profiles depending on the macrostructure of the devices. In the multilayer device incorporating two drugs, the drug release rate was similar for both drugs but faster when the drug loading was higher. In DuoCaplets the drug incorporated in the external layer was released first, and there was a lag time until the release of the drug contained in the core, depending on the characteristics of the external layer. Moreover, the same group [31] used the fused deposition modeling and the hot-melt extrusion to generate paracetamol-loaded tablets from filaments produced from three different grades of hypromellose acetate succinate. The dissolution tests showed that the drug release from the tablets depended on the polymer composition, the drug loading, and the internal structure of the formulations. Especially, all

HPMCAS-based tablets showed initial delayed release in the gastric medium and in the intestinal conditions, and the drug release was faster from the tablets prepared using polymers with a lower pH threshold. These results confirm that the fused deposition modeling 3DP makes possible the production of delayed-release printlets, without the need of enteric coating. Okwuosa et al. [32] managed to fabricate shell-core delayed-release tablets of theophylline, budesonide, and diclofenac sodium with dual fused deposition modeling 3D printing and hot-melt extrusion. For the core structure, filaments consisting of the polymer (PVP), plasticizer (triethyl citrate), filler (talc) or tribasic phosphate sodium, and the active ingredient were created with hot-melt extrusion. While for the shell, Eudragit L100–55, triethyl citrate, and talc were used. The created filaments were then used for the printing of caplets containing the active ingredient in the core, while the shell serves as an enteric coating. This study demonstrated the potential of fabricating patient-specific pH-responsive tablets in one step. In another article, Maroni et al. [33] have reported on the manufacture of a two-compartment capsular device conveying incompatible drugs or differing drug formulations using the fused deposition modeling and injection molding. Through the assembly of compartments that had different wall thickness and/or composition, the drug release could be characterized as pulsatile.

Khaled et al. [34] used the extrusion-based 3DP for the preparation of guaifenesin bilayer tablets with an immediate-release and a sustained-release layer. Drug release kinetics indicated Fickian diffusion drug release through the hydrated HPMC gel layer. The same group of researchers [35] used the same technique for the production of a novel complex geometry "five-in-one" polypill. The drugs, aspirin, hydrochlorothiazide, ramipril, and pravastatin atenolol, were physically separated in the polypill to avoid incompatibility issues and allow maximum flexibility. Release studies revealed immediate and sustained drug release mechanisms.

A research group formulated immediate−/extended-release tablets, which were composed of two drug-containing sections of different pH-based release mechanisms. The pulsed release of the model drug, chlorpheniramine maleate, took place after a lag time of 10 min followed by extended release of the compound over a period of 7 h. Furthermore, enteric dual pulsed-release tablets were constructed and the dissolution profiles showed that two pulses of diclofenac sodium, released, one immediately at t = 1 h and the second pulse began after a lag time of 4 h. The same group of researchers [36] also fabricated dual pulsed-release tablets, where one section eroded immediately in the acidic environment stage releasing diclofenac during the first 30 min, while the second section eroded 5 h later, at higher pH values.

6. Conclusions

The present chapter offers a review of the 3D-printed modified-release oral solid pharmaceutical formulations that have been created up to date. It aims at demonstrating the potential role of this technology in the tailored manufacture of pharmaceutical products. Even though 3DP has been introduced since the 1980s, there is still a lot of exploration in this field, especially for the creation of materials suitable for pharmaceutical and medical applications. One of the ongoing researches in the area is the 3DP of new, versatile materials that have the ability to change their properties under the influence of external factors or over time. The structural modification over time or otherwise called the fourth dimension, created a new term called "4D printing" [37]. In oral dosage forms, this technology allows the modification of drug delivery, since the timely release profile can be triggered by stimuli, such as pH, temperature, enzymes action, and time [38].

Conflict of interest

The authors declare no conflict of interest.

Author details

Angeliki Siamidi, Eleni Tsintavi, Dimitrios M. Rekkas and Marilena Vlachou*
Sector of Pharmaceutical Technology, Department of Pharmacy, School of Health Sciences, National and Kapodistrian University of Athens, Athens, Greece

*Address all correspondence to: vlachou@pharm.uoa.gr

References

[1] Chia HN, Wu BM. Recent advances in 3D printing of biomaterials. Journal of Biological Engineering. 2015;**9**:4. DOI: 10.1186/s13036-015-0001-4

[2] Trenfield SJ, Awad A, Goyanes A, Gaisford S, Basit AW. 3D printing pharmaceuticals: Drug development to frontline care. Trends in Pharmacological Sciences. 2018;**39**(5): 440-451. DOI: 10.1016/j.tips.2018.02.006

[3] Norman J, Madurawe RD, Moore CMV, Khan MA, Khairuzzaman A. A new chapter in pharmaceutical manufacturing: 3D-printed drug products. Advanced Drug Delivery Reviews. 2017;**108**:39-50. DOI: 10.1016/j.addr.2016.03.001

[4] Alhnan MA, Okwuosa TC, Sadia M, Wan KW, Ahmed W, Arafat B. Emergence of 3D printed dosage forms: Opportunities and challenges. Pharmaceutical Research. 2016;**33**(8): 1817-1832. DOI: 10.1007/s11095-016-1933-1

[5] Prasad LK, Smyth H. 3D printing technologies for drug delivery: A review. Drug Development and Industrial Pharmacy. 2015;**42**(7): 1019-1031. DOI: 10.3109/03639045.2015.1120743

[6] Pravin S, Sudhir A. Integration of 3D printing with dosage forms: A new perspective for modern healthcare. Biomedicine and Pharmacotherapy. 2018;**107**:146-154. DOI: 10.1016/j.biopha.2018.07.167

[7] Sandler N, Preis M. Printed drug-delivery systems for improved patient treatment. Trends in Pharmacological Sciences. 2016;**37**(12):1070-1080. DOI: 10.1016/j.tips.2016.10.002

[8] Zema L, Melocchi A, Maroni A, Gazzaniga A. Three-dimensional printing of medicinal products and the challenge of personalized therapy. Journal of Pharmaceutical Sciences. 2017;**106**(7):1697-1705. DOI: 10.1016/j.xphs.2017.03.021

[9] Gibson I, Rosen D, Stucker B. Additive Manufacturing Technologies 3D Printing, Rapid Prototyping, and Direct Digital Manufacturing. New York: Springer-Verlag; 2015. DOI: 10.1007/978-1-4939-2113-3

[10] Goole J, Amighi K. 3D printing in pharmaceutics: A new tool for designing customized drug delivery systems. International Journal of Pharmaceutics. 2016;**499**(1–2):376-394. DOI: 10.1016/j.ijpharm.2015.12.071

[11] Tsintavi E, Rekkas DM, Bettini R. Partial Tablet Coating by 3D Printing. Poster Session Presented at the 3rd European Conference on Pharmaceutics; Bologna, Italy; 2019

[12] Jamróz W, Kurek M, Łyszczarz E, Szafraniec J, Knapik-Kowalczuk J, Syrek K, et al. 3D printed orodispersible films with Aripiprazole. International Journal of Pharmaceutics. 2017;**533**(2): 413-420. DOI: 10.1016/j.ijpharm.2017.05.052

[13] Musazzi UM, Selmin F, Ortenzi MA, Mohammed GK, Franzé S, Minghetti P, et al. Personalized orodispersible films by hot melt ram extrusion 3D printing. International Journal of Pharmaceutics. 2018;**551**(1–2): 52-59. DOI: 10.1016/j.ijpharm.2018.09.013

[14] Kempin W, Domsta V, Grathoff G, Brecht I, Semmling B, Tillmann S, et al. Immediate release 3D-printed tablets produced via fused deposition modeling of a thermo-sensitive drug. Pharmaceutical Research. 2018;**35** (6):124(1-12). DOI: 10.1007/s11095-018-2405-6

[15] Solanki NG, Tahsin M, Shah AV, Serajuddin ATM. Formulation of 3D printed tablet for rapid drug release by fused deposition modeling: Screening polymers for drug release, drug-polymer miscibility and printability. Journal of Pharmaceutical Sciences. 2018;**107**(1):390-401. DOI: 10.1016/j.xphs.2017.10.021

[16] Genina N, Boetker JP, Colombo S, Harmankaya N, Rantanen J, Bohr A. Anti-tuberculosis drug combination for controlled oral delivery using 3D printed compartmental dosage forms: From drug product design to in vivo testing. Journal of Controlled Release. 2017;**268**:40-48. DOI: 10.1016/j.jconrel.2017.10.003

[17] Gioumouxouzis CI, Katsamenis OL, Bouropoulos N, Fatouros DG. 3D printed oral solid dosage forms containing hydrochlorothiazide for controlled drug delivery. Journal of Drug Delivery Science and Technology. 2017;**40**:164-171. DOI: 10.1016/j.jddst.2017.06.008

[18] Goyanes A, Robles Martinez P, Buanz A, Basit AW, Gaisford S. Effect of geometry on drug release from 3D printed tablets. International Journal of Pharmaceutics. 2015;**494**(2):657-663. DOI: 10.1016/j.ijpharm.2015.04.069

[19] Goyanes A, Chang H, Sedough D, Hatton GB, Wang J, Buanz A, et al. Fabrication of controlled-release budesonide tablets via desktop (FDM) 3D printing. International Journal of Pharmaceutics. 2015;**496**(2):414-420. DOI: 10.1016/j.ijpharm.2015.10.039

[20] Goyanes A, Buanz ABM, Hatton GB, Gaisford S, Basit AW. 3D printing of modified-release aminosalicylate (4-ASA and 5-ASA) tablets. European Journal of Pharmaceutics and Biopharmaceutics. 2015;**89**:157-162. DOI: 10.1016/j.ejpb.2014.12.003

[21] Goyanes A, Kobayashi M, Martínez-Pacheco R, Gaisford S, Basit AW. Fused-filament 3D printing of drug products: Microstructure analysis and drug release characteristics of PVA-based caplets. International Journal of Pharmaceutics. 2016;**514**(1):290-295. DOI: 10.1016/j.ijpharm.2016.06.021

[22] Wang J, Goyanes A, Gaisford S, Basit AW. Stereolithographic (SLA) 3D printing of oral modified-release dosage forms. International Journal of Pharmaceutics. 2016;**503**(1–2):207-212. DOI: 10.1016/j.ijpharm.2016.03.016

[23] Yu DG, Yang XL, Huang WD, Liu J, Wang YG, Xu H. Tablets with material gradients fabricated by three-dimensional printing. Journal of Pharmaceutical Sciences. 2007;**96**(9):2446-2456. DOI: 10.1002/jps.20864

[24] Zhang J, Feng X, Patil H, Tiwari RV, Repka MA. Coupling 3D printing with hot-melt extrusion to produce controlled-release tablets. International Journal of Pharmaceutics. 2017;**519**(1–2):186-197. DOI: 10.1016/j.ijpharm.2016.12.049

[25] Pietrzak K, Isreb A, Alhnan MA. A flexible-dose dispenser for immediate and extended release 3D printed tablets. European Journal of Pharmaceutics and Biopharmaceutics. 2015;**96**:380-387. DOI: 10.1016/j.ejpb.2015.07.027

[26] Skowyra J, Pietrzak K, Alhnan MA. Fabrication of extended-release patient-tailored prednisolone tablets via fused deposition modelling (FDM) 3D printing. European Journal of Pharmaceutical Sciences. 2015;**68**:11-17. DOI: 10.1016/j.ejps.2014.11.009

[27] Goyanes A, Buanz ABM, Basit AW, Gaisford S. Fused-filament 3D printing (3DP) for fabrication of tablets. International Journal of Pharmaceutics. 2014;**476**(1–2):88-92. DOI: 10.1016/j.ijpharm.2014.09.044

[28] Kyobula M, Adedeji A, Alexander MR, Saleh E, Wildman R, Ashcroft I, et al. 3D inkjet printing of tablets exploiting bespoke complex geometries for controlled and tuneable drug release. Journal of Controlled Release. 2017;**261**:207-215. DOI: 10.1016/j.jconrel.2017.06.025

[29] Khaled SA, Burley JC, Alexander MR, Yang J, Roberts CJ. 3D printing of tablets containing multiple drugs with defined release profiles. International Journal of Pharmaceutics. 2015;**494**(2):643-650. DOI: 10.1016/j.ijpharm.2015.07.067

[30] Goyanes A, Wang J, Buanz A, Martínez-Pacheco R, Telford R, Gaisford S, et al. 3D printing of medicines: Engineering novel oral devices with unique design and drug release characteristics. Molecular Pharmaceutics. 2015;**12**(11):4077-4084. DOI: 10.1021/acs.molpharmaceut.5b00510

[31] Goyanes A, Fina F, Martorana A, Sedough D, Gaisford S, Basit AW. Development of modified release 3D printed tablets (printlets) with pharmaceutical excipients using additive manufacturing. International Journal of Pharmaceutics. 2017;**527**(1–2):21-30. DOI: 10.1016/j.ijpharm.2017.05.021

[32] Okwuosa TC, Pereira BC, Arafat B, Cieszynska M, Isre A, Alhnan MA. Fabricating a shell-core delayed release tablet using dual FDM3D printing for patient-centred therapy. Pharmaceutical Research. 2017;**34**:427. DOI: 10.1007/s11095-016-2073-3

[33] Maroni A, Melocchi A, Parietti F, Foppoli A, Zema L, Gazzaniga A. 3D printed multi-compartment capsular devices for two-pulse oral drug delivery. Journal of Controlled Release. 2017;**268**:10-18. DOI: 10.1016/j.jconrel.2017.10.008

[34] Khaled SA, Burley JC, Alexander MR, Roberts CJ. Desktop 3D printing of controlled release pharmaceutical bilayer tablets. International Journal of Pharmaceutics. 2014;**461**(1–2):105-111. DOI: 10.1016/j.ijpharm.2013.11.021

[35] Khaled SA, Burley JC, Alexander MR, Yang J, Roberts CJ. 3D printing of five-in-one dose combination polypill with defined immediate and sustained release profiles. Journal of Controlled Release. 2015;**217**:308-314. DOI: 10.1016/j.jconrel.2015.09.028

[36] Rowe C, Katstra W, Palazzolo R, Giritlioglu B, Teung P, Cima M. Multimechanism oral dosage forms fabricated by three dimensional printing™. Journal of Controlled Release. 2000;**66**(1):11-17. DOI: 10.1016/s0168-3659(99)00224-2

[37] Khoo ZX, Teoh JEM, Liu Y, Chua CK, Yang S, An J, et al. 3D printing of smart materials: A review on recent progresses in 4D printing. Virtual and Physical Prototyping. 2015;**10**(3):103-122. DOI: 10.1080/17452759.2015.1097054

[38] Lui YS, Sow WT, Tan LP, Wu Y, Lai Y, Li H. 4D printing and stimuli-responsive materials in biomedical aspects. Acta Biomaterialia. 2019;**92**:19-36. DOI: 10.1016/j.actbio.2019.05.005

Section 3

Structure of Drug-Receptor Complex

Chapter 4

Integrated Molecular Profiling as an Approach to Identify PI3K Inhibitor Resistance Mechanisms

Nicole L. Michmerhuizen, Jiayu Wang and J. Chad Brenner

Abstract

The identification of drug resistance pathways and approaches to target these pathways remains a significant and important challenge in cancer biology. Here, we address this challenge in the context of ongoing efforts to advance phosphatidylinositol 3-kinase (PI3K) inhibitors for the treatment of PI3K-aberrant cancers. While PI3K inhibitors have had tremendous success in some diseases, such as breast cancer, early clinical trials in other malignancies, such as head and neck squamous cell carcinoma (HNSCC), have not had the same level of success. Since HNSCC and other cancers display relatively high PI3K pathway alteration rates (>45%), these underwhelming results suggest that additional or unexpected factors may contribute to the lower response rates. Here, we highlight some of the emerging functional genomic and sequencing approaches being used to identify predictive biomarkers of PI3K inhibitor response using both cancer cell lines and clinical trial specimens. Importantly, these approaches have uncovered both innate genetic and adaptive mechanisms driving PI3K inhibitor resistance. In this chapter, we describe recent technological advances that have revolutionized our understanding of PI3K inhibitor resistance pathways in HNSCC and highlight how these and other approaches lay the groundwork to make significant strides in our understanding of molecular pharmacology in the cancer field.

Keywords: PI3K, targeted therapy, drug combination, drug screening, drug resistance

1. Introduction

Head and neck squamous cell carcinomas (HNSCCs) are malignant neoplasms that can occur in regions including the oral cavity, oropharynx, and larynx. HNSCC is the sixth most common cancer, by incidence, worldwide and constitutes approximately 4% of all cancers globally [1–3]. Tobacco use, alcohol consumption, and/or infection with oncogenic high-risk types of HPV, primarily HPV16, are regarded as the major risk factors for HNSCC [4]. Although traditional treatments for HNSCC include surgery, radiotherapy, and cytotoxic chemotherapy [1], these approaches have only modestly reduced the mortality of HNSCC. In fact, only 40–50% of patients with HNSCC survive for 5 years following diagnosis [5].

2. The phosphatidylinositol 3-kinase (PI3K) pathway in HNSCC

HNSCC sequencing studies have identified highly prevalent PI3K pathway alterations that activate PI3K signaling. Following activation by receptor tyrosine kinases (RTKs) and/or G-protein coupled receptors (GPCRs), PI3K phosphorylates phosphatidylinositol (4,5)-bisphosphate (PIP_2) into an essential second messenger phosphatidylinositol (3,4,5)-trisphosphate (PIP_3) [6]. PIP_3 then recruits and activates proteins like PDK1 and AKT to mediate PI3K's pro-survival functions (**Figure 1A**). As a tumor suppressor, PTEN dephosphorylates PIP_3 into PIP_2 to prevent downstream signal propagation; the deregulation of PTEN is also related to multiple cancers including HNSCC [7].

There are three classes of PI3K (Class I, Class II, and Class III), and Class I PI3K is further divided into Class IA and Class IB [8]. Among the Class IA PI3Ks is p110alpha encoded by the gene *PIK3CA*, which represents the catalytic subunit and alpha isoform of PI3K. Importantly, *PIK3CA* is the most frequently altered gene in the PI3K pathway across all tumors and in HNSCC [9–11]. Alterations of other Class I PI3Ks isoforms, like p110β, and of some regulatory isoforms have been detected in various cancers, albeit with a relatively low frequency [12] (**Figure 2**). Although studies have also examined Class II and Class III PI3Ks, more research is needed to understand their role in human disease [16].

Functionally, the PI3K signaling pathway has a wide range of intracellular effects, including participation in cell cycle, survival, metabolism, motility, and genomic instability [17]. Mutations or other genetic aberrations can lead to hyperactivation of PI3K signaling, and in turn increase cell growth and viability. Angiogenesis and inflammatory cell recruitment, which are thought to be cancer-promoting, may also drive tumor progression and are common in advanced-stage tumors [9, 18].

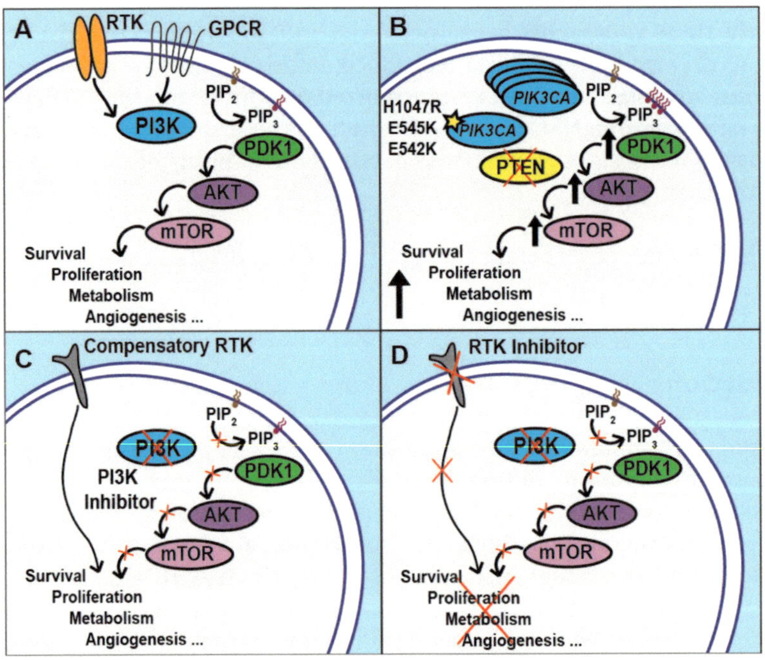

Figure 1.
Rationale for PI3K inhibitor combination therapy. (A) The PI3K signaling pathway has diverse cellular functions. (B) Alterations in PI3K pathway genes may lead to increased signaling. (C) Resistance to PI3K inhibitor monotherapy prevents cell death. (D) Co-targeting PI3K and resistance mechanisms leads to cell death.

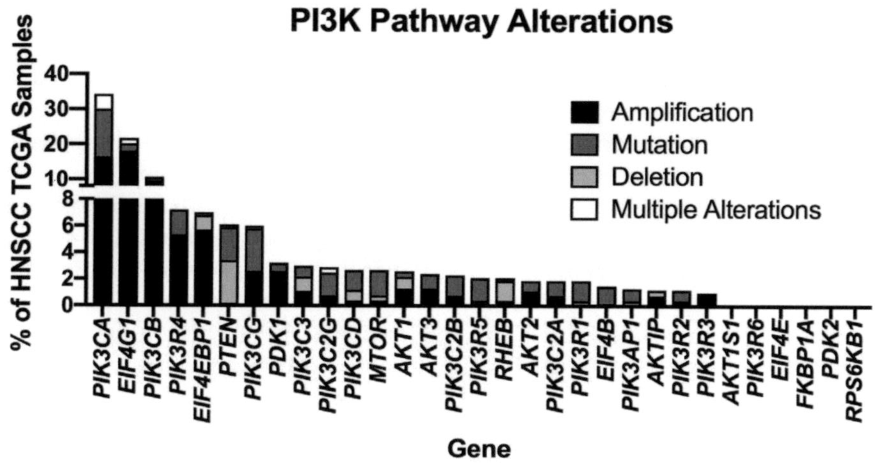

Figure 2.
PI3K pathway gene alteration rates in HNSCC tumors from the cancer genome atlas (TCGA). Amplifications, deletions, mutations and/or multiple alterations (e.g., amplification and mutation) are shown as indicated [13–15].

The first manuscript detailing *PIK3CA* mutations in HNSCC was published in 2006; this study described "hotspot," activating mutations (E542K, E545K, and H1047R) among other *PIK3CA* alterations that are less frequent and have not been as well characterized [19]. Since then, evidence has continued to support the significant role of PI3K signaling in HNSCC. The Cancer Genome Atlas (TCGA) dataset, one of the largest HNSCC sequencing studies performed to date, shows that the PI3K signaling pathway is the most frequently mutated oncogenic and targetable signaling pathway in this cancer type [13, 15, 20]. Additionally, Chung and co-authors independently found that almost 32% of HNSCC patients have *PIK3CA* mutation or copy number alteration after analyzing 252 HNSCC patient samples. This study also indicated that 11% of HPV-positive and 5% of HPV-negative HNSCC patients have loss-of-function mutations or copy number alterations in *PTEN*, the gene responsible for restraining PI3K pathway activation (**Figure 1B**) [21].

The frequency of PI3K pathway alteration suggests that inhibitors targeting this pathway may be of clinical use, and several teams have advanced PI3K inhibitors to test their effectiveness for HNSCC treatment. Early clinical trials demonstrated that PI3K inhibitors were safe for use in patients with solid tumors [22, 23], and studies evaluated the potential benefits of using pan-PI3K-targeting agents in recurrent and metastatic HNSCC specifically. However, PI3K inhibitors have more recently shown limitations in efficacy as well as safety (**Figure 1C**). Jimeno et al. reported in 2015 that pan-PI3K inhibitor PX-866 did not improve outcomes when added to cytotoxic chemotherapy (docetaxel) in unselected recurrent or metastatic (R/M) HNSCC patients [24]. Later, Soulieres and colleagues achieved improvements in overall and progression-free survival when administering another pan-PI3K inhibitor, BKM120, with cytotoxic agent paclitaxel (as compared to paclitaxel alone); this study, the BERIL-1 trial, is discussed further below [25]. Unfortunately, BKM120 has not been evaluated further due to undesired side effects. Current trials are evaluating the clinical effects of other PI3K-targeting drugs (NCT03740100), including those with isoform selectivity (NCT02145312, NCT02822482), in HNSCC patients.

The lack of patient selection is one potential contributor to the underwhelming efficacy of PI3K inhibitor treatment in HNSCCs to date. Although the majority of TCGA HNSCC patients display aberration in one or more PI3K pathway genes [14], the status of any single gene or any group of genes has not been validated as a critical biomarker of response to PI3K inhibition. This is in contrast to recent data for hormone receptor-positive breast cancer, where PI3K inhibitor alpelisib is used in combination with fulvestrant to prolong survival for patients with *PIK3CA* mutant tumors [26]. While precision medicine trials across a variety of cancer types have also shown a trend supporting *PIK3CA* alterations as a marker for response to PI3K inhibitors [27], *PIK3CA* mutation has not yet been associated with sensitivity to PI3K inhibition in HNSCC trials [24, 28]. Studies evaluating the role of *PIK3CA* mutations in response to PI3K inhibition in HNSCC often do not reach statistical significance or have a very limited number of patients enrolling. For example, Janku et al. conducted an analysis of responses to PI3K/AKT/mTOR inhibitors in tumors with H1047R *PIK3CA* mutations including four HNSCC patients; after inhibitor treatment, two of these patients experienced progressive disease, one had little change in tumor burden, and another had an incomplete response to therapy [29]. It is possible that the difference in outcomes between tumors with and without *PIK3CA* mutations has not been noted due to an insufficient number of *PIK3CA* mutant tumors in any single clinical trial. Ongoing studies of PI3K inhibitor copanlisib in HNSCC patients with *PIK3CA* mutation or amplification or *PTEN* loss will better elucidate any potential differences in response attributable to PI3K activation (NCT02822482). It is also feasible that other features predict responses to PI3K inhibitor. In the recent BERIL-1 study, which compared outcomes in R/M HNSCC patients (n = 79 per group) treated with paclitaxel with or without pan-PI3K inhibitor BKM120, follow-up analysis revealed that *TP53* alteration, low tumor mutation burden, HPV negativity, and high infiltration of tumor infiltrating lymphocytes (TILs) or CD8+ T-cells was associated with improved response to BKM120. Recent preclinical work has proposed that loss-of-function mutations in *NOTCH1* may predict response to PI3K inhibition [30]. Together these data suggest that a more nuanced understanding of tissue type-specific factors and PI3K inhibitor response mechanisms may be required to develop clinically effective companion diagnostics for this class of inhibitors in HNSCC.

Our recent report indicates that responses to PI3K inhibition, either as monotherapy or in combination with other targeted inhibitors, are complex and cannot be predicted solely based on genetic mutation, copy number alteration, or RNA expression of a single gene (submitted). In this study, a diverse set of HNSCC cell lines were treated with PI3K inhibitors of varying isoform selectivity as monotherapies. Alpha isoform-targeting agents were clearly more effective than other PI3K inhibitors, but the sensitivity profiles for any individual pan- or alpha-isoform PI3K inhibitor were more difficult to stratify. This was increasingly true when PI3K inhibitors were used in drug combinations: *PIK3CA* mutation, copy number, RNA expression, and HPV status did not prove to be meaningful biomarkers for either PI3K and epidermal growth factor receptor (EGFR) inhibitor dual-therapies [31] or for other synergistic drug pairs. In the case of PI3Kalpha inhibitor HS-173 and FAK inhibitor TAE226, greater synergy was observed in *PIK3CA* mutant cell lines as compared to *PIK3CA* wildtype cell lines in initial validation experiments. However, when this association was tested more rigorously with other PI3K and FAK inhibitors, dual-therapy was beneficial also in many *PIK3CA* wildtype models; this could be due to differences in selectivity or mechanism of action for individual small molecule drugs [32]. Thus, PI3K pathway activation, measured at the DNA level via mutation or copy number status or at the protein level via relative downstream phosphorylation, appears to be an insufficient biomarker for sensitivity in HNSCC cell lines; other cellular features, including additional alteration in PI3K pathway members (such as downstream mutations in *AKT1*) or activation of receptor tyrosine kinases (perhaps via upstream overexpression of EGFR), may contribute to signaling through the PI3K pathway and thereby affect inhibitor responses. Indeed, multifaceted analyses, such as those considering gene sets rather than individual genetic changes, may be needed to predict sensitivity. For example, responses to EGFR or FAK inhibitor may be better stratified using gene sets incorporating activation of PI3K, mTOR, or other related signaling nodes instead of *PIK3CA* mutation status alone. Alternatively, an additional pathway that is changed as a result of PI3K activation (e.g., epithelial to mesenchymal transition, cell cycle, or apoptosis) may be even more effective in predicting response.

More broadly, activation or blockade of PI3K signaling may impact response to other forms of cancer treatment. Clinical trial data have not demonstrated that mutation, amplification, or loss of PI3K pathway genes is linked to sensitivity or resistance to PI3K inhibitors. However, recent trials for EGFR-targeting agents have noted poorer outcomes following EGFR inhibition in patients with PI3K activation. In the phase III E2303 trial, which compared cisplatin with or without cetuximab in without cetuximab in R/M HNSCC patients [33], *PIK3CA* mutation or *PTEN* loss was associated with poor response to EGFR-targeting therapy [34]. This finding was also noted in the LUX-H&N1 trial, which compared second-line treatments with afatinib and methotrexate in R/M HNSCCs [35]; here, tumors lacking *PTEN* received inferior benefit from afatinib as compared to those with high levels of *PTEN* [36]. Preclinical studies have also noted that PI3K activation or *PTEN* loss may serve as a biomarker for resistance to cetuximab [37, 38] and that *PIK3CA* mutant HNSCC models may be more resistant to cyclin-dependent kinase (CDK) inhibitor palbociclib [39]. Further studies are warranted to validate these results in larger, prospective trials.

3. Combination drug strategies may overcome compensatory PI3K inhibitor resistance

3.1 Epidermal growth factor receptor (EGFR)

One of the most widely studied mechanisms of resistance to PI3K inhibition is signaling through members of the ERBB family, primarily EGFR, and the downstream Ras-MEK-ERK effector pathway. The human ERBB gene family encodes four members of the ERBB family of receptors including EGFR/ERBB1/HER1, NEU/ERBB2/HER2, ERBB3/HER3 and ERBB4/HER4. As a transmembrane receptor, EGFR can be activated by ligands including epidermal growth factor (EGF). EGFR signaling subsequently activates downstream pathways, including RAS-RAF-MEK-ERK. MAPK and PI3K-AKT-mTOR signaling pathways, to promote cell proliferation and inhibit apoptosis in many head and neck models [40, 41]. EGFR overexpression has been reported in the vast majority of HNSCCs [42]. Further genetic dysregulations of EGFR signaling caused by *EGFR* gene mutation (although rare in head and neck cancer) and *EGFR* gene copy number amplification (approximately 10% of cases) also contribute to activated EGFR signaling [41, 43].

Activation of EGFR signaling as a mechanism of PI3K inhibitor resistance has been extensively characterized using a wide variety of cell lines (displaying a diverse array of genetic alterations) and a large set of ERBB family-targeting drugs [1, 31, 44–47]. Early work focused on *PIK3CA*-amplified HNSCCs demonstrated that two-thirds (67%) of cell lines with additional copies of wildtype *PIK3CA* maintained RAS-RAF-MEK-ERK MAPK pathway activity following PI3K inhibitor treatment and that two of these models were also sensitive to dual inhibition of PI3K and EGFR or MEK [1]. A more recent publication extended this observation to a larger panel of ERBB inhibitors and cell lines, including several with *PIK3CA* mutations [31]. Overall, findings from the latter study mirrored those of previous publications showing that dual-therapy with PI3K and EGFR inhibitors was often more effective than either monotherapy [44–47], but also extended this observation to consider individual classes of ERBB-targeting agents that might result in heightened responses when used as part of combination treatments. Results in HNSCC cell lines showed that *irreversible* inhibitors of EGFR were more effective in combination with PI3K inhibitors than reversible ERBB-targeting agents. As previous work had primarily considered dual-therapies that included either reversible EGFR inhibitors or EGFR-targeting antibodies such as cetuximab, this work was the first direct comparison of PI3K inhibitors in combination with distinct pharmacologies against EGFR.

Beyond direct inhibition of the receptor tyrosine kinases PI3K and EGFR themselves, previous work has also examined drug combinations targeting PI3K and EGFR via inhibition of downstream effectors including mTOR and MEK, respectively. Several papers have described synergy with mTOR inhibitors and EGFR agents [48–50]. In one of these studies, Jimeno et al. used H1047R *PIK3CA* mutant Detroit 562 cells in a xenograft model and noted improved response to mTOR inhibitor temsirolimus and erlotinib. This response co-occurred with changes in MAPK and p70 S6 kinase phosphorylation (downstream of EGFR and mTOR, respectively) and in Ki67, effects that were not evidenced in less responsive xenograft models or after single-agent treatment. Other work with Detroit 562 in vitro showed minimal responses to PI3K inhibitor HS-173 and reversible EGFR inhibitors, including erlotinib, that could be enhanced to synergistic levels with multiple irreversible EGFR inhibitors [31]. The combination of erlotinib with mTOR inhibitors (temsirolimus or otherwise) has not been reported in this model. Nevertheless, since additional data show that ineffective reversible EGFR inhibitor combinations block MAPK phosphorylation [31] (p70 S6 kinase phosphorylation was not tested), it is possible that one or more additional effectors, perhaps further downstream of MAPK/p70 S6 kinase or as part of a second escape pathway, may be responsible for synergistic effects. Alternatively, in vitro and in vivo responses to mTOR and EGFR agents in Detroit 562 and potentially other HNSCCs could be dependent on distinct mechanisms. PI3K and irreversible EGFR inhibitor combinations have not yet been tested in xenografts, but these experiments would enhance our understanding of the potential for such dual-therapies to translate clinically.

In light of the synergy observed following treatment with agents targeting the PI3K and EGFR pathways in preclinical models, phase I and II trials have been performed to examine these dual-therapies in HNSCC patients. Of these trials, three have been completed, all in patients receiving second-line treatment due to chemotherapy resistance, recurrence, and/or metastasis. The first of these trials examined temsirolimus with cetuximab and resulted in dose-limited toxicities in one-third of patients [51]. The second considered another mTOR inhibitor, everolimus, with erlotinib. This combination had a reasonable toxicity profile and stopped or decreased tumor growth in several patients, but it did not result in clinical benefit as compared to previous trials considering erlotinib as a monotherapy [52]. The third trial, which considered cetuximab with or without PI3K inhibitor PX-866, also did not provide evidence of improvement with the addition of PI3K inhibitor [53]. Several other trials using PI3K- and EGFR-targeting agents, sometimes alongside cytotoxic chemotherapy or radiotherapy, have been initiated and are in various stages of completion. Toxicity seems to be a major concern in many of these studies and may limit the use of such combinations in patients. As a result, the development of more specific combinations is warranted.

Nevertheless, previous work also suggests that the use of currently available PI3K and EGFR therapies may be optimized in other ways. For example, the sequence of combination treatments may be an important consideration. Lattanzio et al. showed that Cal-33 cells responded to treatment with EGFR antibody followed by PI3K inhibitor [54], while other data show minimal responses in this model when EGFR- and PI3K-targeting small molecules were co-administered [31]. The type of EGFR-targeting agent that was used may also explain this conflicting data: small molecules (e.g., gefitinib, erlotinib, afatinib) and biologics (e.g., cetuximab) could have very different response profiles in combination with PI3K inhibitors.

Overall, although responses to PI3K and EGFR inhibitor combinations in HNSCC have been studied more extensively than many other dual-therapies for this cancer type, current results highlight the diversity of responses to agents targeting these two signaling pathways. Additional factors, including but not limited to timing, patient selection, and other co-treatments, require further consideration before compensation through the PI3K and EGFR pathways will be most effectively exploited in a population of HNSCC patients.

3.2 Other ERBB family members

Additional studies have successfully implicated other means of upstream inhibition in combination with PI3K-targeting drugs to improve responses in HNSCC, including other members of the ERBB family. While the structure of these members is similar to that of EGFR, each ERBB receptor has a different ligand binding specificity and physiological role [55]. Abnormalities of ERBB2, ERBB3, and ERBB4 have been reported in various malignancies such as breast cancer and occur in smaller subsets of head and neck cancer; therefore, they also became the targets for cancer therapies and have been considered in drug combinations [55, 56].

For example, Brand and co-authors blocked ERBB3 signaling as a means of reversing PI3K inhibitor resistance mediated by HPV oncoproteins E6 and E7 in HPV-positive HNSCCs [57]. These studies support the role of RTKs in HNSCC resistance mechanisms and validate that combination PI3K and RTK blockade may result in improved PI3K inhibitor responses. Likewise, Meister et al. also reported that PI3K inhibition induces ERBB3 upregulation and activation while the combination of PI3K and ERBB3 inhibition has synergistic effect, suppressing HNSCC growth both in vitro and in vivo [58]. Furthermore, in breast cancer, researchers also found that amplification of *ERBB2* can activate PI3K-AKT signaling directly and indirectly [59], and ERBB2 inhibition potentiates the antitumor effect of PI3K inhibitor BEZ235 in this cancer type [60].

3.3 AXL receptor tyrosine kinase

PI3K inhibitor resistance mechanisms, of course, span far beyond the ERBB family of RTKs alone. For instance, the AXL receptor tyrosine kinase is highly expressed in various cancers including esophageal squamous cell carcinoma and HNSCC [61]. Based on work by Elkabets et al., AXL is upregulated particularly in PI3K inhibitor-resistant HNSCCs [62]. These researchers also showed that the dimerization of AXL and EGFR promotes signaling through PI3K and mTOR by activating the PLCγ-PKC signaling pathway, thereby limiting the efficacy of PI3K inhibitors. This PI3K-independent activation of mTOR counteracts the growth inhibitory effect of PI3K inhibition and mediates drug resistance in some head and neck models [62]. Further, Badarni et al. chose to identify and target the transcription factors that were responsible for the increased expression of AXL in HNSCCs. In doing so, they discovered that a c-JUN, a member of the AP-1 transcription factor (TF) complex, was likely responsible for AXL upregulation and that blocking this TF improved the response to PI3K inhibitor BYL719 [63].

3.4 Insulin-like growth factor-1 receptor (IGF-1R)

IGFR signaling is vital in the development of tissues [64] and is aberrantly implicated in several types of cancer including adenomas, breast cancer, lung cancer, ovarian cancer, and HNSCC [65]. *IGF1R* is amplified in 4% of HNSCC tumors from TCGA, placing it among the most commonly amplified genes in this tumor type [13–15]. Both IGF-1R and IGF binding protein-3 (IGFBP-3) have overt impact on HNSCC prognoses, as clinical data reveal that high expression of IGFBP-3 as well as the co-expression of IGFBP-3 with IGF-1R may predict poor prognosis in this cancer type [66]. Preclinical models also demonstrate the role of the IGF-1R signaling pathway in HNSCC: small molecule IGF-1R inhibitor BMS-536924 is effective in both cell lines derived from transgenic mice that spontaneously developed salivary gland tumors and in xenograft mouse models [67].

The tyrosine kinase activity of IGF-1R suggests that the activation of IGF-1R could induce activation of PI3K signaling [68, 69]. Interestingly, studies suggest that the activation of mTOR signaling could be part of a negative feedback loop to reduce PI3K signaling by the phosphorylation of insulin receptor substrate-1 (IRS-1) [70]. This complex relationship between the PI3K and IGFR signaling pathways indicates that IGFR signaling could be a compensatory mechanism contributing to PI3K inhibitor resistance, a phenomenon that has been previously observed in multiple other cancer types [71, 72]. Recent data (submitted) also indicate the potential efficacy of PI3K and IGF-1R inhibitor combinations in HNSCC models, but such dual-therapies have yet to be evaluated in patients.

3.5 Anaplastic lymphoma kinase (ALK)

Aberration in the *ALK* gene is associated with several cancer types; gene fusions have been noted in anaplastic large cell lymphoma and one subset of non-small cell lung cancer [73], while mutations are present in nearly 15% of neuroblastomas [74]. ALK has also been shown to have a pleiotropic role in the aggressive growth and invasiveness of oral squamous cell carcinoma [75]. As a downstream member of the ALK signaling pathway, PI3K/AKT signaling may be activated followed by ALK activation [76]. Collectively, these data motivate consideration of ALK signaling as a compensatory signaling pathway responsible for resistance to PI3K inhibitor monotherapies.

ALK signaling has not historically been evaluated as a resistance mechanism in HNSCC, since fusion events are rare and ALK expression is often quite low in this cancer type. Nevertheless, recent work has shown that EGFR inhibitor treatments may increase the expression of ALK and display greater efficacy with ALK inhibitors [77, 78]. Gonzales et al. showed that the combination of ALK inhibitor and EGFR inhibitor could decrease HNSCC cell proliferation in vitro as well as reduce the volumes of xenotransplantation tumors in vivo [77]. These studies demonstrate that ALK signaling is indeed an important mediator of drug resistance in some head and neck cancers. Additionally, *ALK* was also identified in a CRISPR/Cas9 knockout screen as one of the kinases responsible for resistance to PI3K inhibitor treatment (submitted). PI3K and ALK dual-therapy, however, has not been considered in HNSCC. The only previous studies of PI3K and ALK inhibitors examine such combinations in the context of other tumor types driven by ALK signaling due to fusion with *EML4* or other genes [79–82]. Our recent work shows that co-treatment with ALK inhibitor brigatinib and PI3K inhibitor pictilisib is synergistic in HNSCC models (submitted); this may represent the first evidence of interaction between PI3K and ALK signaling in the absence of *ALK* gene fusion.

However, brigatinib is not a perfectly selective inhibitor of ALK—it also displays activity at IGF-1R, EGFR, and other RTKs, especially at higher concentrations [83, 84]. While ALK inhibition may be an important component of the response to combinations of brigatinib and PI3K inhibitor, we cannot exclude the possibility that the blockade of IGF-1R and/or EGFR contribute at least partially to this response. Both small molecule profiling studies and subsequent validation analyses show that IGF-1R or EGFR inhibition can improve responses to PI3K-targeting therapy, as noted above. Genetic knockouts of *ALK* and *IGF1R* that were generated in combination-responsive HSC-4 cells offer insight into the effect of blocking an individual RTK, mimicking a perfectly selective pharmacologic treatment. *ALK* knockout HSC-4 cells are more sensitive to monotherapy with AKT inhibitor GDC-0068 than wildtype HSC-4 cells. Responses to PI3K inhibition are not markedly different in the knockout model, suggesting that ALK alone may not be responsible for the synergy of ALK- and PI3K-targeting agents in HNSCC. In spite of this, *ALK* and *IGF1R* knockout cell lines display increased levels of p110alpha, the protein encoded by the *PIK3CA* gene (submitted). This indicates an important molecular relationship between the ALK, IGF-1R, and PI3K pathways and may explain the lack of response to PI3K inhibition in knockout cell lines.

While the mechanistic basis for responses to pictilisib and brigatinib has not been fully elucidated, co-treatment with these agents three times per week inhibited tumor growth in a cell line-derived xenograft mouse model (submitted). However, despite the significant result observed after a 3-week course with these inhibitors, tumors did progress as treatment continued for extended lengths of time. This observation is in support of the development of additional compensatory mechanisms mediating treatment resistance. Although the combination of PI3K and ALK inhibitor extended survival for weeks past what would have been observed in mice with vehicle- and brigatinib-treated tumors, further exploration of compensatory signaling in HNSCC and the development of improved treatment paradigms is needed.

3.6 Fibroblast growth factor receptor (FGFR)

FGFRs also have been nominated as a critical candidate for compensatory signaling pathway in HNSCC. After the binding of the fibroblast growth factor (FGF) ligands, the FGFR signaling pathway will modify downstream phosphorylation and gene expression. Importantly, this pathway also has a well-described role in HNSCC pathogenesis due to recurrent of genetic alterations that occur in the disease [85]. According to previous studies, recurrent FGFR1 amplification is present in 17% of OSCC cases [86]. A high level of FGFR2 expression, FGFR3 expression and FGFR2/FGFR3 co-expression are also observed in HNSCC cell lines [87], and such alterations have been suggested to contribute to the early stages of tumor initiation and disease progression [88]. In fact, previous in vitro and in vivo studies show that inhibition of the FGFR signaling pathway could decrease the proliferation of HNSCC supporting cells (fibroblast and endothelial cells) and ultimately results in a decline of tumor cell proliferation through increased cell apoptosis [89]. Combinations of EGFR and FGFR inhibitors have been evaluated in both HNSCC and other cancers, most notably lung cancer [90, 91], but have not translated to the clinic due to toxic effects in patients [92]. Based on these and other data demonstrating the important role of FGFR signaling in HNSCC [93], combinations of PI3K and FGFR inhibitors might be synergistic in a subset of patients.

3.7 Focal adhesion kinase (FAK)

Although most pathways nominated as drivers of PI3K inhibitor resistance are RTKs, a potential relationship between PI3K and the cytoplasmic FAK receptor has also been described. FAK, which is encoded by the Protein Tyrosine Kinase 2 (*PTK2*) gene [94], has a wide range of intracellular functions, involving regulation of cell adhesion, cell proliferation, migration, and cell apoptosis, all of which are commonly altered in head and neck cancer [95]. One previous study assessed 147 HNSCC clinical tumor samples and reported FAK protein overexpression and *PTK2* gene amplification in 62 and 39% of these samples, respectively, supporting a molecular role for this kinase in HNSCC [96]. FAK inhibitors serve to arrest the cell cycle and decrease tumor cell viability via the induction of apoptosis [97]. One such inhibitor, TAE226, is able to induce the tumor cell apoptosis and in turn suppress HNSCC growth in vitro; this inhibitor also blocked tumor growth, metastasis, and angiogenesis in vivo [98]. The mechanisms by which the FAK signaling pathway is involved in tumor cell metastases and growth may be kinase-dependent; in this case, FAK is upstream of PI3K signaling pathway. One hypothesis is that activation of FAK could induce the PI3K and subsequent downstream signaling including remodeling of the cytoskeletal, matrix metalloproteinases (MMPs) as well as formation or turnover of focal adhesion. Such effects might contribute to the metastases of tumor cells. Activation of the FAK-PI3K signaling pathway has also been shown to inhibit tumor cell apoptosis [99–102]. Interestingly, loss of *PTEN*, has been shown to stimulate FAK and downstream targets [103]. However, a role for FAK inhibition has not been well described in cases of *PIK3CA* amplification or mutation. One clinical trial (NCT02372227) sought to evaluate the safety of combining PI3K and FAK inhibitors VS-5584 and VS-6063 in malignant mesothelioma but was terminated prior to completion. A recent report (submitted) shows that FAK/IGF-1R inhibitor TAE226 may be synergistic with PI3K inhibitors in HNSCC cell lines and xenografts, but the contribution of FAK signaling and the mechanism for this effect have yet to be fully determined. Taken together, however, this collection of data nominates FAK signaling as a means of resistance to PI3K inhibitor monotherapy in HNSCC.

3.8 Aurora kinase A (AURKA)

Aurora kinase A (AURKA) is another player identified as having a potentially indispensable role in PI3K inhibitor response in some HNSCCs. AURKA is one of the aurora serine-threonine kinase family members, which play an important role in the regulation of cell cycle and cell division by controlling mitosis and meiosis [104]. In normal cells, AURKA regulates mitosis by contributing to maturation of the centrosome, synthesizing of bipolar spindle, and controlling cytokinesis. Researchers also showed that the upregulation of AURKA is associated with worse prognosis and decreased survival of patients with HNSCCs [105–107]. These poor outcomes are postulated to result from associated centrosome abnormalities and chromosomal aneusomy as well as activation of the spindle assembly checkpoint [106, 108]. AURKA is also involved in both AKT and FAK signaling pathways, and this AURKA/AKT/FAK signaling axis can be responsible for the migration and invasion of HNSCCs [109]. Previous research shows that suppression of AURKA via shRNA could inhibit the ability of laryngeal carcinoma cells to grow and invade both in vitro and in vivo, suggesting that AURKA inhibitor monotherapy may have a substantial effect on oncogenic phenotypes in some models [110]. Furthermore, recent data (submitted) indicate that the regulation of cell cycle gene expression and protein levels, including AURKA, is reduced by synergistic PI3K inhibitor dual-therapies. The altered function of AURKA shows that aurora kinases could play a pivotal compensatory signaling role in PI3K inhibitor resistance.

3.9 Cell apoptosis

Overactivation of PI3K/AKT pathway can inhibit tumor cell apoptosis and promote cell proliferation. The family of forkhead transcription factors (FOXOs) is among the specific downstream PI3K/AKT effectors involved in the regulation of cell apoptosis. The PI3K/AKT pathway mediates serine/threonine phosphorylation of FOXO transcription factors, which reverses the pro-apoptotic effect of FOXOs by downregulating the pro-apoptotic protein BIM, a Bcl-2 family member. Conversely, the use of PI3K and AKT inhibitors may induce cell apoptosis in various tumor types, a phenomenon already detailed in breast cancer models [111]. PI3K/AKT inhibition reduces FOXO phosphorylation leading to the upregulation of BIM [112], an effect that may contribute to apoptosis. The role of specific FOXO family members and their transcriptional targets as well as how these functions are altered by modulation of PI3K signaling has yet to be fully determined in HNSCC.

3.10 PDK1, AKT, and mTOR

Much of the previous work on compensatory resistance to PI3K inhibition has noted contributions from pathways downstream of PI3K or other codependent RTKs, including PDK1 [30], AKT [113], mTOR [114–116], and MEK [117, 118]. Previous publications [117, 118] show that inhibiting PI3K and MEK is functionally similar to inhibiting PI3K and EGFR (see above). Prior studies have also highlighted the importance of PI3K effector AKT in combination responses; these publications describe similar evidence of synergy when replacing PI3K inhibitors with AKT inhibition or siRNA [46] and report reduced AKT phosphorylation following combination PI3K and EGFR inhibitor treatments [44, 46, 47, 82, 119]. Similarly, the work of Sambandam et al. demonstrates the importance of PDK1 inhibition in PI3K inhibitor responses by showing that: (1) reductions in the level of phosphorylated and total PDK1 were present in cell lines that were more sensitive to PI3K inhibition and (2) AKT inhibitor MK-2206 and PDK1 inhibitor GSK2334470 were synergistic when used together, recapitulating or exceeding the effects of PI3K inhibitor monotherapy [30]. In contrast, other analyses (submitted) demonstrate that AKT phosphorylation was similarly reduced following treatment with PI3K monotherapy and ineffective combinations as compared to treatment with synergistic drug pairs. This may suggest that AKT inhibition is necessary, but not sufficient, for response to PI3K inhibitor therapy. PDK1 phosphorylation was also unchanged with PI3K mono- and dual-therapy in this recent dataset (submitted), and little benefit was noted with PDK1, AKT, or mTOR inhibitors to PI3K inhibitors. Based on these findings, it seems that although PDK1, AKT, and mTOR are downstream effectors common to PI3K and the other RTKs involved in synergistic drug pairs, additional mechanisms are responsible for combination effects.

Clinical data evaluating the contribution of targeting both PI3K and its downstream PI3K remain immature. Trials have been performed to determine the safe dose of PI3K inhibitor BEZ235 in combination with mTOR inhibitors RAD001 (NCT01482156) or everolimus (NCT01508104), but results have yet to be published. While there is a trial of PI3K/mTOR inhibitor bimiralisib (NCT03740100) currently ongoing, the contribution of PI3K and mTOR individually will be impossible to ascertain from this study alone.

3.11 Immunotherapy

Emerging data suggest that the PI3K pathway may interact with immune responses and improve the efficacy of immune checkpoint receptor (ICR) blockade. One indication of the involvement of the PI3K pathway in responses to immunotherapies is based on data using models with loss of tumor suppressor *PTEN*. In multiple cancer types, increased expression of programmed death ligand-1 (PD-L1) has been observed in models with loss of *PTEN* [120–123], and there is some evidence that this may also be the case in HNSCC [124].

PI3K signaling also may interface with immune responses through its important role in cellular metabolism. In cancerous cells, the metabolic balance shifts from oxidative phosphorylation to aerobic glycolysis as part of a paradigm known as the Warburg effect [17]. A notable consequence of this effect is the inefficient use of glucose, which limits the maximum possible amount of ATP or energy. Since PI3K pathway activity contributes to glucose uptake and glycolysis [125], cancer cells displaying PI3K pathway activation (through *PIK3CA* mutation, *PTEN* loss or other genetic or functional changes) may utilize additional glucose from the tumor microenvironment. Nearby cytotoxic T-lymphocytes (CTLs) and other immunomodulatory cells, which require vast amounts of glucose to launch and maintain effective immune attack on tumor spread, are therefore in heated competition with PI3K pathway-activated cells for the limited glucose supply. As such, CTL activation, including migration to the tumor site, production of cytokines, and other immune functions, is limited and CTL exhaustion occurs more rapidly [126–130]. PI3K inhibition, however, alters cellular metabolism to prevent or delay CTL exhaustion and thereby allows for a faster and/or more durable CTL response.

Additionally, PI3K inhibition may enhance the effects of ICR blockade by preventing adaptive resistance. One mechanism that may blunt responses to ICR blockade involves the compensatory upregulation of other ICRs. Shayan and coworkers showed that in HNSCC tumor samples, two ICRs, programmed cell death receptor-1 (PD-1) and T-cell Ig and mucin domain-3 protein (TIM-3), were co-expressed on CTLs displaying high levels of exhaustion [131]. PD-1 blockade resulted in further upregulation of TIM-3; this upregulation was reversible using PI3K inhibition [131]. Thus, through multiple means, PI3K inhibition may augment responses to immunotherapy in HNSCC. Clinical trials to evaluate therapies that combine PI3K inhibitor and ICR blockade are ongoing (including NCT04317105 to evaluate PD-1 inhibitor nivolumab and PI3K inhibitor copanlisib in solid tumors), and the results of these studies will offer critical insights for the future of targeted and immunotherapies in HNSCC and other cancers.

4. Conclusions

Due to advances in diverse profiling strategies ranging from next generation sequencing to combinatorial high throughput small molecule profiling to pooled CRISPR and shRNA screens, recent technological advances have led to significant scientific advances in understanding the mechanisms that drive response to PI3K inhibitors in HNSCC and other cancers. Indeed, the future is bright for the advancement of PI3K inhibitors, especially as combination therapies, in HNSCC and other cancer types. Nevertheless, multiple questions remain regarding the role of specific signaling pathways in PI3K inhibitor resistance, and additional studies will be required to further our understanding of this important intersection of pharmacology and cancer biology. More work is needed to develop safer, more effective drugs, to establish biomarkers for response, and to target critical resistance mechanisms. The studies described in this chapter serve as a contribution in these efforts. With the combined efforts of the community, PI3K inhibitors may, in time, have a place among standard-of-care treatments for HNSCC.

Conflict of interest

The authors declare no conflict of interest.

Author details

Nicole L. Michmerhuizen[1,2], Jiayu Wang[1,2] and J. Chad Brenner[1,2,3,4]*

1 Department of Otolaryngology – Head and Neck Surgery, University of Michigan Medical School, Ann Arbor, MI, United States

2 Department of Pharmacology, University of Michigan Medical School, Ann Arbor, MI, United States

3 Program in Cellular and Molecular Biology, University of Michigan Medical School, Ann Arbor, MI, United States

4 Rogel Cancer Center, University of Michigan Medical School, Ann Arbor, MI, United States

*Address all correspondence to: chadbren@umich.edu

References

[1] Michmerhuizen NL, Leonard E, Kulkarni A, Brenner JC. Differential compensation mechanisms define resistance to PI3K inhibitors in PIK3CA amplified HNSCC. Otorhinolaryngology-Head and Neck Surgery. 2016;**1**(2):44-50

[2] Sanderson R, Wei WI, Ironside J. Clinical review: Squamous cell carcinomas of the head and neck. Commentary: Head and neck carcinomas in the developing world. BMJ. 2002;**325**(7368):822-827

[3] Vigneswaran N, Williams MD. Epidemiologic trends in head and neck cancer and aids in diagnosis. Oral and Maxillofacial Surgery Clinics. 2014;**26**(2):123-141

[4] Marur S, D'Souza G, Westra WH, Forastiere AA. HPV-associated head and neck cancer: A virus-related cancer epidemic. The Lancet Oncology. 2010;**11**(8):781-789

[5] Leemans CR, Braakhuis BJ, Brakenhoff RH. The molecular biology of head and neck cancer. Nature Reviews. Cancer. 2011;**11**(1):9

[6] Fruman DA, Chiu H, Hopkins BD, Bagrodia S, Cantley LC, Abraham RT. The PI3K pathway in human disease. Cell. 2017;**170**(4):605-635

[7] Papa A, Pandolfi PP. The PTEN(-) PI3K axis in cancer. Biomolecules. 2019;**9**(4):153

[8] Liu P, Cheng H, Roberts TM, Zhao JJ. Targeting the phosphoinositide 3-kinase pathway in cancer. Nature Reviews. Drug Discovery. 2009;**8**(8):627-644

[9] Velho PI, Castro G, Chung CH. Targeting the PI3K pathway in head and neck squamous cell carcinoma. American Society of Clinical Oncology Educational Book. 2015;**35**:123-128

[10] Lui VW, Hedberg ML, Li H, Vangara BS, Pendleton K, Zeng Y, et al. Frequent mutation of the PI3K pathway in head and neck cancer defines predictive biomarkers. Cancer Discovery. 2013;**3**(7):761-769

[11] Fruman DA, Rommel C. PI3K and cancer: Lessons, challenges and opportunities. Nature Reviews. Drug Discovery. 2014;**13**(2):140

[12] Thorpe LM, Yuzugullu H, Zhao JJ. PI3K in cancer: Divergent roles of isoforms, modes of activation and therapeutic targeting. Nature Reviews. Cancer. 2015;**15**(1):7-24

[13] Gao J, Aksoy BA, Dogrusoz U, Dresdner G, Gross B, Sumer SO, et al. Integrative analysis of complex cancer genomics and clinical profiles using the cBioPortal. Science Signaling. 2013;**6**(269):pl1

[14] Cancer Genome Atlas Network. Comprehensive genomic characterization of head and neck squamous cell carcinomas. Nature. 2015;**517**(7536):576-582

[15] Cerami E, Gao J, Dogrusoz U, Gross BE, Sumer SO, Aksoy BA, et al. The cBio cancer genomics portal: An open platform for exploring multidimensional cancer genomics data. Cancer Discovery. 2012;**2**(5):401-404

[16] Jean S, Kiger AA. Classes of phosphoinositide 3-kinases at a glance. Journal of Cell Science 2014;127(Pt 5): 923-928

[17] Hanahan D, Weinberg RA. Hallmarks of cancer: The next generation. Cell. 2011;**144**(5):646-674

[18] Osaki M, Oshimura M, Ito H. PI3K-Akt pathway: Its functions and alterations in human cancer. Apoptosis. 2004;**9**(6):667-676

[19] Qiu W, Schonleben F, Li X, Ho DJ, Close LG, Manolidis S, et al. PIK3CA mutations in head and neck squamous cell carcinoma. Clinical Cancer Research: An Official Journal of the American Association for Cancer Research. 2006;**12**(5):1441-1446

[20] Cai Y, Dodhia S, Su GH. Dysregulations in the PI3K pathway and targeted therapies for head and neck squamous cell carcinoma. Oncotarget. 2017;**8**(13):22203

[21] Chung CH, Guthrie VB, Masica DL, Tokheim C, Kang H, Richmon J, et al. Genomic alterations in head and neck squamous cell carcinoma determined by cancer gene-targeted sequencing. Annals of Oncology: Official Journal of the European Society for Medical Oncology. 2015;**26**(6):1216-1223

[22] Bendell JC, Rodon J, Burris HA, de Jonge M, Verweij J, Birle D, et al. Phase I, dose-escalation study of BKM120, an oral pan-class I PI3K inhibitor, in patients with advanced solid tumors. Journal of Clinical Oncology: Official Journal of the American Society of Clinical Oncology. 2012;**30**(3):282-290

[23] Ando Y, Inada-Inoue M, Mitsuma A, Yoshino T, Ohtsu A, Suenaga N, et al. Phase I dose-escalation study of Buparlisib (BKM120), an oral pan-class I PI3K inhibitor, in Japanese patients with advanced solid tumors. Cancer Science. 2014;**105**(3):347-353

[24] Jimeno A, Bauman JE, Weissman C, Adkins D, Schnadig I, Beauregard P, et al. A randomized, phase 2 trial of docetaxel with or without PX-866, an irreversible oral phosphatidylinositol 3-kinase inhibitor, in patients with relapsed or metastatic head and neck squamous cell cancer. Oral Oncology. 2015;**51**(4):383-388

[25] Soulieres D, Faivre S, Mesia R, Remenar E, Li SH, Karpenko A, et al. Buparlisib and paclitaxel in patients with platinum-pretreated recurrent or metastatic squamous cell carcinoma of the head and neck (BERIL-1): A randomised, double-blind, placebo-controlled phase 2 trial. The Lancet Oncology. 2017;**18**(3):323-335

[26] Andre F, Ciruelos E, Rubovszky G, Campone M, Loibl S, Rugo HS, et al. Alpelisib for PIK3CA-mutated, hormone receptor-positive advanced breast cancer. The New England Journal of Medicine. 2019;**380**(20):1929-1940

[27] Chau NG, Li YY, Jo VY, Rabinowits G, Lorch JH, Tishler RB, et al. Incorporation of next-generation sequencing into routine clinical care to direct treatment of head and neck squamous cell carcinoma. Clinical Cancer Research: An Official Journal of the American Association for Cancer Research. 2016;**22**(12):2939-2949

[28] Soulieres D, Licitra L, Mesia R, Remenar E, Li SH, Karpenko A, et al. Molecular alterations and Buparlisib efficacy in patients with squamous cell carcinoma of the head and neck: Biomarker analysis from BERIL-1. Clinical Cancer Research: An Official Journal of the American Association for Cancer Research. 2018;**24**(11):2505-2516

[29] Janku F, Wheler JJ, Naing A, Falchook GS, Hong DS, Stepanek VM, et al. PIK3CA mutation H1047R is associated with response to PI3K/AKT/mTOR signaling pathway inhibitors in early-phase clinical trials. Cancer Research. 2013;**73**(1):276-284

[30] Sambandam V, Frederick MJ, Shen L, Tong P, Rao X, Peng S, et al. PDK1 mediates NOTCH1-mutated head and neck squamous carcinoma vulnerability to therapeutic PI3K/mTOR inhibition. Clinical Cancer Research: An Official Journal of the American Association for Cancer Research. 1 Jun 2019;**25**(11):3329-3340

[31] Michmerhuizen NL, Leonard E, Matovina C, Harris M, Herbst G, Kulkarni A, et al. Rationale for using

irreversible epidermal growth factor receptor inhibitors in combination with phosphatidylinositol 3-kinase inhibitors for advanced head and neck squamous cell carcinoma. Molecular Pharmacology. 2019;**95**(5):528-536

[32] Liu TJ, LaFortune T, Honda T, Ohmori O, Hatakeyama S, Meyer T, et al. Inhibition of both focal adhesion kinase and insulin-like growth factor-I receptor kinase suppresses glioma proliferation in vitro and in vivo. Molecular Cancer Therapeutics. 2007;**6**(4):1357-1367

[33] Burtness B, Goldwasser MA, Flood W, Mattar B, Forastiere AA. Phase III randomized trial of cisplatin plus placebo compared with cisplatin plus cetuximab in metastatic/recurrent head and neck cancer: An Eastern Cooperative Oncology Group study. Journal of Clinical Oncology: Official Journal of the American Society of Clinical Oncology. 2005;**23**(34):8646-8654

[34] Psyrri A, Lee JW, Pectasides E, Vassilakopoulou M, Kosmidis EK, Burtness BA, et al. Prognostic biomarkers in phase II trial of cetuximab-containing induction and chemoradiation in resectable HNSCC: Eastern cooperative oncology group E2303. Clinical Cancer Research: An Official Journal of the American Association for Cancer Research. 2014;**20**(11):3023-3032

[35] Machiels JP, Haddad RI, Fayette J, Licitra LF, Tahara M, Vermorken JB, et al. Afatinib versus methotrexate as second-line treatment in patients with recurrent or metastatic squamous-cell carcinoma of the head and neck progressing on or after platinum-based therapy (LUX-Head & Neck 1): An open-label, randomised phase 3 trial. The Lancet Oncology. 2015;**16**(5):583-594

[36] Cohen EEW, Licitra LF, Burtness B, Fayette J, Gauler T, Clement PM, et al. Biomarkers predict enhanced clinical outcomes with afatinib versus methotrexate in patients with second-line recurrent and/or metastatic head and neck cancer. Annals of Oncology: Official Journal of the European Society for Medical Oncology. 2017;**28**(10):2526-2532

[37] Eze N, Lee JW, Yang DH, Zhu F, Neumeister V, Sandoval-Schaefer T, et al. PTEN loss is associated with resistance to cetuximab in patients with head and neck squamous cell carcinoma. Oral Oncology. 2019;**91**:69-78

[38] Keysar SB, Astling DP, Anderson RT, Vogler BW, Bowles DW, Morton JJ, et al. A patient tumor transplant model of squamous cell cancer identifies PI3K inhibitors as candidate therapeutics in defined molecular bins. Molecular Oncology. 2013;7(4):776-790

[39] Zainal NS, Lee BKB, Wong ZW, Chin IS, Yee PS, Gan CP, et al. Effects of palbociclib on oral squamous cell carcinoma and the role of PIK3CA in conferring resistance. Cancer Biology & Medicine. 2019;**16**(2):264-275

[40] Singh B, Carpenter G, Coffey RJ. EGF receptor ligands: Recent advances. F1000Research. 2016;**5**(F1000 Faculty Rev):2270

[41] Wee P, Wang Z. Epidermal growth factor receptor cell proliferation signaling pathways. Cancers (Basel). 2017;**9**(5):52

[42] Ozanne B, Richards CS, Hendler F, Burns D, Gusterson B. Over-expression of the EGF receptor is a hallmark of squamous cell carcinomas. The Journal of Pathology. 1986;**149**(1):9-14

[43] Gazdar AF. Activating and resistance mutations of EGFR in non-small-cell lung cancer: Role in clinical response to EGFR tyrosine kinase inhibitors. Oncogene. 2009;**28**(Suppl 1):S24-S31

[44] Rebucci M, Peixoto P, Dewitte A, Wattez N, De Nuncques MA, Rezvoy N, et al. Mechanisms underlying resistance to cetuximab in the HNSCC cell line: Role of AKT inhibition in bypassing this resistance. International Journal of Oncology. 2011;**38**(1):189-200

[45] Anisuzzaman AS, Haque A, Wang D, Rahman MA, Zhang C, Chen Z, et al. In vitro and in vivo synergistic antitumor activity of the combination of BKM120 and erlotinib in head and neck cancer: Mechanism of apoptosis and resistance. Molecular Cancer Therapeutics. 2017;**16**(4):729-738

[46] Silva-Oliveira RJ, Melendez M, Martinho O, Zanon MF, de Souza Viana L, Carvalho AL, et al. AKT can modulate the in vitro response of HNSCC cells to irreversible EGFR inhibitors. Oncotarget. 2017;**8**(32):53288-53301

[47] Young NR, Liu J, Pierce C, Wei TF, Grushko T, Olopade OI, et al. Molecular phenotype predicts sensitivity of squamous cell carcinoma of the head and neck to epidermal growth factor receptor inhibition. Molecular Oncology. 2013;**7**(3):359-368

[48] Wang Z, Martin D, Molinolo AA, Patel V, Iglesias-Bartolome R, Degese MS, et al. mTOR co-targeting in cetuximab resistance in head and neck cancers harboring PIK3CA and RAS mutations. Journal of the National Cancer Institute. 2014;**106**(9):dju215

[49] Jimeno A, Kulesza P, Wheelhouse J, Chan A, Zhang X, Kincaid E, et al. Dual EGFR and mTOR targeting in squamous cell carcinoma models, and development of early markers of efficacy. British Journal of Cancer. 2007;**96**(6):952-959

[50] Bozec A, Ebran N, Radosevic-Robin N, Sudaka A, Monteverde M, Toussan N, et al. Combination of mTOR and EGFR targeting in an orthotopic xenograft model of head and neck cancer. The Laryngoscope. 2016;**126**(4):E156-E163

[51] Bauman JE, Arias-Pulido H, Lee SJ, Fekrazad MH, Ozawa H, Fertig E, et al. A phase II study of temsirolimus and erlotinib in patients with recurrent and/or metastatic, platinum-refractory head and neck squamous cell carcinoma. Oral Oncology. 2013;**49**(5):461-467

[52] Massarelli E, Lin H, Ginsberg LE, Tran HT, Lee JJ, Canales JR, et al. Phase II trial of everolimus and erlotinib in patients with platinum-resistant recurrent and/or metastatic head and neck squamous cell carcinoma. Annals of Oncology: Official Journal of the European Society for Medical Oncology. 2015;**26**(7):1476-1480

[53] Jimeno A, Shirai K, Choi M, Laskin J, Kochenderfer M, Spira A, et al. A randomized, phase II trial of cetuximab with or without PX-866, an irreversible oral phosphatidylinositol 3-kinase inhibitor, in patients with relapsed or metastatic head and neck squamous cell cancer. Annals of Oncology: Official Journal of the European Society for Medical Oncology. 2015;**26**(3):556-561

[54] Lattanzio L, Tonissi F, Monteverde M, Vivenza D, Russi E, Milano G, et al. Treatment effect of buparlisib, cetuximab and irradiation in wild-type or PI3KCA-mutated head and neck cancer cell lines. Investigational New Drugs. 2015;**33**(2):310-320

[55] Wieduwilt MJ, Moasser MM. The epidermal growth factor receptor family: Biology driving targeted therapeutics. Cellular and Molecular Life Sciences: CMLS. 2008;**65**(10):1566-1584

[56] Mishra R, Patel H, Alanazi S, Yuan L, Garrett JT. HER3 signaling and targeted therapy in cancer. Oncology Reviews. 2018;**12**(1):355

[57] Brand TM, Hartmann S, Bhola NE, Li H, Zeng Y, O'Keefe RA,

et al. Cross-talk signaling between HER3 and HPV16 E6 and E7 mediates resistance to PI3K inhibitors in head and neck cancer. Cancer Research. 2018;**78**(9):2383-2395

[58] Meister KS, Godse NR, Khan NI, Hedberg ML, Kemp C, Kulkarni S, et al. HER3 targeting potentiates growth suppressive effects of the PI3K inhibitor BYL719 in pre-clinical models of head and neck squamous cell carcinoma. Scientific Reports. 2019;**9**(1):9130

[59] Ruiz-Saenz A, Dreyer C, Campbell MR, Steri V, Gulizia N, Moasser MM. HER2 amplification in tumors activates PI3K/Akt signaling independent of HER3. Cancer Research. 2018;**78**(13):3645-3658

[60] Serra V, Scaltriti M, Prudkin L, Eichhorn PJ, Ibrahim YH, Chandarlapaty S, et al. PI3K inhibition results in enhanced HER signaling and acquired ERK dependency in HER2-overexpressing breast cancer. Oncogene. 2011;**30**(22):2547-2557

[61] Rankin EB, Giaccia AJ. The receptor tyrosine kinase AXL in cancer progression. Cancers. 2016;**8**(11):103

[62] Elkabets M, Pazarentzos E, Juric D, Sheng Q, Pelossof RA, Brook S, et al. AXL mediates resistance to PI3Kalpha inhibition by activating the EGFR/PKC/mTOR axis in head and neck and esophageal squamous cell carcinomas. Cancer Cell. 2015;**27**(4):533-546

[63] Badarni M, Prasad M, Balaban N, Zorea J, Yegodayev KM, Ben-Zion J, et al. Repression of AXL expression by AP-1/JNK blockage overcomes resistance to PI3Ka therapy. JCI Insight. 2019;5(8):e125341

[64] Limesand KH, Chibly AM, Fribley A. Impact of targeting insulin-like growth factor signaling in head and neck cancers. Growth Hormone & IGF Research. 2013;**23**(5):135-140

[65] Denduluri SK, Idowu O, Wang Z, Liao Z, Yan Z, Mohammed MK, et al. Insulin-like growth factor (IGF) signaling in tumorigenesis and the development of cancer drug resistance. Genes & Diseases. 2015;**2**(1):13-25

[66] Sun J-M, Jun HJ, Ko YH, Park YH, Ahn YC, Son Y-I, et al. Insulin-like growth factor binding protein-3, in association with IGF-1 receptor, can predict prognosis in squamous cell carcinoma of the head and neck. Oral Oncology. 2011;**47**(8):714-719

[67] Lara PC, Bordón E, Rey A, Moreno M, Lloret M, Henríquez-Hernández LA. IGF-1R expression predicts clinical outcome in patients with locally advanced oral squamous cell carcinoma. Oral Oncology. 2011;**47**(7):615-619

[68] Shepherd PR, Withers DJ, Siddle K. Phosphoinositide 3-kinase: The key switch mechanism in insulin signalling. The Biochemical Journal 1998;333(3):471-490

[69] Roith DL. The insulin-like growth factor system. Experimental Diabetes Research. 2003;**4**(4):205-212

[70] Oliveira JC, Souza KK, Dias MM, Faria MC, Ropelle ER, Flores MB, et al. Antineoplastic effect of rapamycin is potentiated by inhibition of IRS-1 signaling in prostate cancer cells xenografts. Journal of Cancer Research and Clinical Oncology. 2008;**134**(8):833-839

[71] Zorea J, Prasad M, Cohen L, Li N, Schefzik R, Ghosh S, et al. IGF1R upregulation confers resistance to isoform-specific inhibitors of PI3K in PIK3CA-driven ovarian cancer. Cell Death & Disease. 2018;**9**(10):944

[72] Leroy C, Ramos P, Cornille K, Bonenfant D, Fritsch C, Voshol H, et al. Activation of IGF1R/p110beta/AKT/mTOR confers resistance to

alpha-specific PI3K inhibition. Breast Cancer Research: BCR. 2016;**18**(1):41

[73] Mologni L. Inhibitors of the anaplastic lymphoma kinase. Expert Opinion on Investigational Drugs. 2012;**21**(7):985-994

[74] Trigg RM, Turner SD. ALK in neuroblastoma: Biological and therapeutic implications. Cancers. Apr 2018;**10**(4):113

[75] Huang T-T, Gonzales CB, Gu F, Hsu Y-T, Jadhav RR, Wang C-M, et al. Epigenetic deregulation of the anaplastic lymphoma kinase gene modulates mesenchymal characteristics of oral squamous cell carcinomas. Carcinogenesis. 2013;**34**(8):1717-1727

[76] Solomon B, Wilner K, Shaw A. Current status of targeted therapy for anaplastic lymphoma kinase-rearranged non-small cell lung cancer. Clinical Pharmacology and Therapeutics. 2014;**95**(1):15-23

[77] Gonzales CB, De La Chapa JJ, Saikumar P, Singha PK, Dybdal-Hargreaves NF, Chavez J, et al. Co-targeting ALK and EGFR parallel signaling in oral squamous cell carcinoma. Oral Oncology. 2016;**59**:12-19

[78] Ouyang X, Barling A, Lesch A, Tyner JW, Choonoo G, Zheng C, et al. Induction of anaplastic lymphoma kinase (ALK) as a novel mechanism of EGFR inhibitor resistance in head and neck squamous cell carcinoma patient-derived models. Cancer Biology & Therapy. 2018;**19**(10):921-933

[79] Redaelli S, Ceccon M, Zappa M, Sharma GG, Mastini C, Mauri M, et al. Lorlatinib treatment elicits multiple on- and off-target mechanisms of resistance in ALK-driven cancer. Cancer Research. 2018;**78**(24):6866-6880

[80] Tsuji T, Ozasa H, Aoki W, Aburaya S, Funazo T, Furugaki K, et al. Alectinib resistance in ALK-rearranged lung cancer by dual salvage signaling in a clinically paired resistance model. Molecular Cancer Research: MCR. 2019;**17**(1):212-224

[81] Moore NF, Azarova AM, Bhatnagar N, Ross KN, Drake LE, Frumm S, et al. Molecular rationale for the use of PI3K/AKT/mTOR pathway inhibitors in combination with crizotinib in ALK-mutated neuroblastoma. Oncotarget. 2014;**5**(18):8737-8749

[82] Yang L, Li G, Zhao L, Pan F, Qiang J, Han S. Blocking the PI3K pathway enhances the efficacy of ALK-targeted therapy in EML4-ALK-positive nonsmall-cell lung cancer. Tumour Biology. 2014;**35**(10):9759-9767

[83] Huang WS, Liu S, Zou D, Thomas M, Wang Y, Zhou T, et al. Discovery of Brigatinib (AP26113), a phosphine oxide-containing, potent, orally active inhibitor of anaplastic lymphoma kinase. Journal of Medicinal Chemistry. 2016;**59**(10):4948-4964

[84] Uchibori K, Inase N, Araki M, Kamada M, Sato S, Okuno Y, et al. Brigatinib combined with anti-EGFR antibody overcomes osimertinib resistance in EGFR-mutated non-small-cell lung cancer. Nature Communications. 2017;**8**:14768

[85] Dailey L, Ambrosetti D, Mansukhani A, Basilico C. Mechanisms underlying differential responses to FGF signaling. Cytokine & Growth Factor Reviews. 2005;**16**(2):233-247

[86] Freier K, Schwaenen C, Sticht C, Flechtenmacher C, Mühling J, Hofele C, et al. Recurrent FGFR1 amplification and high FGFR1 protein expression in oral squamous cell carcinoma (OSCC). Oral Oncology. 2007;**43**(1):60-66

[87] Marshall ME, Hinz TK, Kono SA, Singleton KR, Bichon B, Ware KE, et al. Fibroblast growth factor receptors are components of autocrine signaling networks in head and neck squamous

cell carcinoma cells. Clinical Cancer Research. 2011;**17**(15):5016-5025

[88] Vairaktaris E, Ragos V, Yapijakis C, Derka S, Vassiliou S, Nkenke E, et al. FGFR-2 and-3 play an important role in initial stages of oral oncogenesis. Anticancer Research. 2006;**26**(6B): 4217-4221

[89] Sweeny L, Liu Z, Lancaster W, Hart J, Hartman YE, Rosenthal EL. Inhibition of fibroblasts reduced head and neck cancer growth by targeting fibroblast growth factor receptor. The Laryngoscope. 2012;**122**(7):1539-1544

[90] Koole K, Brunen D, van Kempen PM, Noorlag R, de Bree R, Lieftink C, et al. FGFR1 is a potential prognostic biomarker and therapeutic target in head and neck squamous cell carcinoma. Clinical Cancer Research: An Official Journal of the American Association for Cancer Research. 2016;**22**(15):3884-3893

[91] Quintanal-Villalonga A, Molina-Pinelo S, Cirauqui C, Ojeda-Marquez L, Marrugal A, Suarez R, et al. FGFR1 cooperates with EGFR in lung cancer oncogenesis, and their combined inhibition shows improved efficacy. Journal of Thoracic Oncology: Official Publication of the International Association for the Study of Lung Cancer. 2019;**14**(4):641-655

[92] Das M, Padda SK, Frymoyer A, Zhou L, Riess JW, Neal JW, et al. Dovitinib and erlotinib in patients with metastatic non-small cell lung cancer: A drug-drug interaction. Lung Cancer (Amsterdam, Netherlands). 2015;**89**(3):280-286

[93] Chae YK, Pai SG, Sun P, Costa R, Matsangou M, Agulnik M, et al. Fibroblast growth factor receptor (FGFR) as a therapeutic target in lung and head and neck cancer. American Journal of Hematology/Oncology®. 2016;**12**(3):13-19

[94] André E, Beckerandre M. Expression of an N-terminally truncated form of human focal adhesion kinase in brain. Biochemical and Biophysical Research Communications. 1993;**190**(1):140-147

[95] Golubovskaya VM. Focal adhesion kinase as a cancer therapy target. Anti-Cancer Agents in Medicinal Chemistry (Formerly Current Medicinal Chemistry-Anti-Cancer Agents). 2010;**10**(10):735-741

[96] Canel M, Secades P, Rodrigo J-P, Cabanillas R, Herrero A, Suarez C, et al. Overexpression of focal adhesion kinase in head and neck squamous cell carcinoma is independent of FAK gene copy number. Clinical Cancer Research. 2006;**12**(11):3272-3279

[97] Tai Y-L, Chen L-C, Shen T-L. Emerging roles of focal adhesion kinase in cancer. BioMed Research International. 2015;**2015**:1-13

[98] Kurio N, Shimo T, Fukazawa T, Okui T, Hassan NMM, Honami T, et al. Anti-tumor effect of a novel FAK inhibitor TAE226 against human oral squamous cell carcinoma. Oral Oncology. 2012;**48**(11):1159-1170

[99] Chen J-S, Huang X-h, Wang Q, Huang J-Q, L-j Z, Chen X-L, et al. Sonic hedgehog signaling pathway induces cell migration and invasion through focal adhesion kinase/AKT signaling-mediated activation of matrix metalloproteinase (MMP)-2 and MMP-9 in liver cancer. Carcinogenesis. 2012;**34**(1):10-19

[100] Zhao J, Guan J-L. Signal transduction by focal adhesion kinase in cancer. Cancer Metastasis Reviews. 2009;**28**(1-2):35-49

[101] Reif S, Lang A, Lindquist JN, Yata Y, Gäbele E, Scanga A, et al. The role of focal adhesion kinase-phosphatidylinositol 3-kinase-akt

signaling in hepatic stellate cell proliferation and type I collagen expression. The Journal of Biological Chemistry. 2003;**278**(10):8083-8090

[102] Sulzmaier FJ, Jean C, Schlaepfer DD. FAK in cancer: Mechanistic findings and clinical applications. Nature Reviews. Cancer. 2014;**14**(9):598

[103] Alfieri R, Giovannetti E, Bonelli M, Cavazzoni A. New treatment opportunities in phosphatase and Tensin homolog (PTEN)-deficient tumors: Focus on PTEN/focal adhesion kinase pathway. Frontiers in Oncology. 2017;**7**:170

[104] Crane R, Gadea B, Littlepage L, Wu H, Ruderman JV. Aurora A, meiosis and mitosis. Biology of the Cell. 2004;**96**(3):215-229

[105] Mehra R, Serebriiskii IG, Burtness B, Astsaturov I, Golemis EA. Aurora kinases in head and neck cancer. The Lancet Oncology. 2013;**14**(10):e425-ee35

[106] Marumoto T, Zhang D, Saya H. Aurora-A—A guardian of poles. Nature Reviews. Cancer. 2005;**5**(1):42

[107] Reiter R, Gais P, Jütting U, Steuer-Vogt MK, Pickhard A, Bink K, et al. Aurora kinase A messenger RNA overexpression is correlated with tumor progression and shortened survival in head and neck squamous cell carcinoma. Clinical Cancer Research. 2006;**12**(17):5136-5141

[108] Anand S, Penrhyn-Lowe S, Venkitaraman AR. AURORA-A amplification overrides the mitotic spindle assembly checkpoint, inducing resistance to Taxol. Cancer Cell. 2003;**3**(1):51-62

[109] Wu J, Yang L, Shan Y, Cai C, Wang S, Zhang H. AURKA promotes cell migration and invasion of head and neck squamous cell carcinoma through regulation of the AURKA/Akt/FAK signaling pathway. Oncology Letters. 2016;**11**(3):1889-1894

[110] Zhang H, Chen X, Liu B, Zhou L. Effects of stable knockdown of Aurora kinase A on proliferation, migration, chromosomal instability, and expression of focal adhesion kinase and matrix metalloproteinase-2 in HEp-2 cells. Molecular and Cellular Biochemistry. 2011;**357**(1-2):95-106

[111] Will M, Qin ACR, Toy W, Yao Z, Rodrik-Outmezguine V, Schneider C, et al. Rapid induction of apoptosis by PI3K inhibitors is dependent upon their transient inhibition of RAS-ERK signaling. Cancer Discovery. 2014;**4**(3):334-347

[112] Urbich C, Knau A, Fichtlscherer S, Walter DH, Brühl T, Potente M, et al. FOXO-dependent expression of the proapoptotic protein Bim: Pivotal role for apoptosis signaling in endothelial progenitor cells. The FASEB Journal. 2005;**19**(8):974-976

[113] Erlich RB, Kherrouche Z, Rickwood D, Endo-Munoz L, Cameron S, Dahler A, et al. Preclinical evaluation of dual PI3K-mTOR inhibitors and histone deacetylase inhibitors in head and neck squamous cell carcinoma. British Journal of Cancer. 2012;**106**(1):107-115

[114] Tonlaar N, Galoforo S, Thibodeau BJ, Ahmed S, Wilson TG, Yumpo Cardenas P, et al. Antitumor activity of the dual PI3K/MTOR inhibitor, PF-04691502, in combination with radiation in head and neck cancer. Radiotherapy and Oncology. 2017;**124**(3):504-512

[115] Elkabets M, Vora S, Juric D, Morse N, Mino-Kenudson M, Muranen T, et al. mTORC1 inhibition is required for sensitivity to PI3K p110alpha inhibitors in PIK3CA-mutant breast cancer. Science Translational Medicine. 2013;**5**(196):196ra99

[116] Ruicci KM, Pinto N, Khan MI, Yoo J, Fung K, MacNeil D, et al. ERK-TSC2 signalling in constitutively-active HRAS mutant HNSCC cells promotes resistance to PI3K inhibition. Oral Oncology. 2018;**84**:95-103

[117] Mohan S, Vander Broek R, Shah S, Eytan DF, Pierce ML, Carlson SG, et al. MEK inhibitor PD-0325901 overcomes resistance to PI3K/mTOR inhibitor PF-5212384 and potentiates antitumor effects in human head and neck squamous cell carcinoma. Clinical Cancer Research: An Official Journal of the American Association for Cancer Research. 2015;**21**(17):3946-3956

[118] Mazumdar T, Byers LA, Ng PK, Mills GB, Peng S, Diao L, et al. A comprehensive evaluation of biomarkers predictive of response to PI3K inhibitors and of resistance mechanisms in head and neck squamous cell carcinoma. Molecular Cancer Therapeutics. 2014;**13**(11):2738-2750

[119] Benavente S, Huang S, Armstrong EA, Chi A, Hsu KT, Wheeler DL, et al. Establishment and characterization of a model of acquired resistance to epidermal growth factor receptor targeting agents in human cancer cells. Clinical Cancer Research: An Official Journal of the American Association for Cancer Research. 2009;**15**(5):1585-1592

[120] Xu C, Fillmore CM, Koyama S, Wu H, Zhao Y, Chen Z, et al. Loss of Lkb1 and Pten leads to lung squamous cell carcinoma with elevated PD-L1 expression. Cancer Cell. 2014;**25**(5):590-604

[121] Zhu J, Chen L, Zou L, Yang P, Wu R, Mao Y, et al. MiR-20b, -21, and -130b inhibit PTEN expression resulting in B7-H1 over-expression in advanced colorectal cancer. Human Immunology. 2014;**75**(4):348-353

[122] Zhang Y, Zhang J, Xu K, Xiao Z, Sun J, Xu J, et al. PTEN/PI3K/mTOR/B7-H1 signaling pathway regulates cell progression and immuno-resistance in pancreatic cancer. Hepato-Gastroenterology. 2013;**60**(127):1766-1772

[123] Parsa AT, Waldron JS, Panner A, Crane CA, Parney IF, Barry JJ, et al. Loss of tumor suppressor PTEN function increases B7-H1 expression and immunoresistance in glioma. Nature Medicine. 2007;**13**(1):84-88

[124] Lyford-Pike S, Peng S, Young GD, Taube JM, Westra WH, Akpeng B, et al. Evidence for a role of the PD-1:PD-L1 pathway in immune resistance of HPV-associated head and neck squamous cell carcinoma. Cancer Research. 2013;**73**(6):1733-1741

[125] Courtnay R, Ngo DC, Malik N, Ververis K, Tortorella SM, Karagiannis TC. Cancer metabolism and the Warburg effect: The role of HIF-1 and PI3K. Molecular Biology Reports. 2015;**42**(4):841-851

[126] Sugiura A, Rathmell JC. Metabolic barriers to T cell function in tumors. Journal of Immunology. 2018;**200**(2):400-407

[127] Siska PJ, Rathmell JC. T cell metabolic fitness in antitumor immunity. Trends in Immunology. 2015;**36**(4):257-264

[128] Delgoffe GM, Powell JD. Feeding an army: The metabolism of T cells in activation, anergy, and exhaustion. Molecular Immunology. 2015;**68**(2 Pt C):492-496

[129] Topalian SL, Taube JM, Anders RA, Pardoll DM. Mechanism-driven biomarkers to guide immune checkpoint blockade in cancer therapy. Nature Reviews. Cancer. 2016;**16**(5):275-287

[130] Palucka AK, Coussens LM. The basis of oncoimmunology. Cell. 2016;**164**(6):1233-1247

[131] Shayan G, Srivastava R, Li J, Schmitt N, Kane LP, Ferris RL. Adaptive resistance to anti-PD1 therapy by Tim-3 upregulation is mediated by the PI3K-Akt pathway in head and neck cancer. Oncoimmunology. 2017;**6**(1):e1261779

Chapter 5

Allosteric Modulators for GPCRs as a Therapeutic Alternative with High Potential in Drug Discovery

Arfaxad Reyes Alcaraz, Emilio Y. Lucero Garcia-Rojas, Richard A. Bond and Bradley K. McConnell

Abstract

The superfamily of G protein-coupled receptors (GPCRs) consists of biological microprocessors that can activate multiple signaling pathways. Most GPCRs have an orthosteric pocket where the endogenous ligand(s) typically binds. Conversely, allosteric ligands bind to GPCRs at sites that are distinct from the orthosteric binding region and they modulate the response elicited by the endogenous ligand. Allosteric ligands can also switch the response of a GPCR after ligand binding to a unique signaling pathway, these ligands are termed biased allosteric modulators. Thus, the development of allosteric ligands opens new and multiple ways in which the signaling pathways of GPCRs can be manipulated for potential therapeutic benefit. Furthermore, the mechanisms by which allosteric ligands modulate the effects of endogenous ligands have provided new insights into the interactions between allosteric ligands and GPCRs. These new findings have a high potential to improve drug discovery and development and, therefore, creating the need for better screening methods for allosteric drugs to increase the chances of success in the development of allosteric modulators as lead clinical compounds.

Keywords: GPCRs, allosteric modulators, biased signaling, β-Arrestin, G-protein, orthosteric site, endogenous agonist

1. Introduction

Allosteric modulators are small molecules or peptides that by specifically interacting with the receptor can alter the affinity, and/or efficacy of the endogenous hormone or other orthosteric ligands including antagonists, and possibly even constitutive signaling by GPCRs. By modifying these pharmacological parameters, allosteric modulators can exert multiple effects on the signaling of GPCRs. Positive Allosteric Modulators (PAMs) potentiate the signaling of the receptor by increasing the affinity and/or efficacy of the endogenous ligand or other administered agonists. On the contrary, Negative Allosteric Modulators (NAMs) decrease the affinity and/or efficacy of the agonists. Biased Allosteric Modulators (BAMs) will direct the agonist response to a single signaling pathway [1, 2].

Before going deeper into pharmacological concepts, it is necessary to define fundamental parameters used to describe the activity of a ligand. Affinity refers to the capacity of a ligand to bind to a receptor. The efficacy of a ligand, is the ability of a ligand to activate or amplify a response after binding to a receptor. Then Furchgott defined intrinsic efficacy as efficacy divided by the total receptor number, in hopes of defining a unique ligand-receptor value much like a ligand's affinity [3]. Earlier, Ariens had introduced the term 'intrinsic activity' of a ligand to explain the behavior of partial agonists [4]. Ariens proposed assigning the maximum response of the endogenous ligand a value of 1 or 100% and partial agonists were expressed as a fraction of this response. The discovery of inverse agonists, ligands that can shut down constitutive signaling by a GPCR expanded the scale from −1 to 1 (or − 100–100%). A ligand that does not produce a cellular response (i.e., zero efficacy) when bound to the orthosteric site of the receptor is termed an antagonist [5].

The site to which endogenous agonists bind to is defined as the orthosteric site. Allosteric modulators do not bind to this site. They bind to other sites and are thus termed allosteric sites [6]. Upon binding, modulators generally stabilize a pre-existing conformation or change the structural conformation of the receptor. This will often modulate the orthosteric site and can modify the effects of the agonists, or in theory, inverse agonists [1]. Allosteric modulators can also stabilize one of the multiple conformational states of the receptor [7].

Experimentally, allosteric modulation can be challenging because the allosteric modulators may affect the affinity and/or efficacy differently for each agonist (see agonist or probe dependence discussed below). For instance, different agonists that induce the same cellular response, after binding to the same receptor, can be differentially modulated by the same allosteric modulator [1]. Furthermore, they are usually difficult to screen for because they do not produce an effect by themselves and may not displace radiolabeled ligands used in binding assays.

Drugs that target the orthosteric site of G protein-coupled receptors (GPCRs) are currently the most common therapeutic tools. Allosteric binding sites (e.g., sites elsewhere on the receptors) are less well-defined and, therefore, less exploited clinically. Diversity in location, mechanism, and specificity of allosteric ligands are characteristics giving them a great potential to extend the range of the ways that drugs can modulate GPCR signaling.

2. Advantages of allosteric modulators

Allosteric modulators with no intrinsic efficacy will usually only exert their effects in the presence of an endogenous agonist. Thus, they can selectively tune cellular responses in tissues where the endogenous agonist exerts its physiological or pathophysiological functions. As a result, temporal and spatial aspects of the endogenous agonist signaling can be chronically maintained or even corrected in pathological states. Also, the saturation of allosteric binding sites limits itself the action of the allosteric modulator and the effect on the function of the agonist. This excellent property of the agonist overcomes the overdosing of a drug, making the allosteric modulators much safer than classical drugs [8].

A great benefit of using allosteric ligands for therapeutic applications is their huge potential to achieve greater selectivity at subtypes of GPCRs [8]. This could be due to greater diversity in the amino acid sequence of the allosteric binding sites compared to the orthosteric binding pocket. Another possibility is via selective cooperativity between the allosteric and orthosteric binding sites at a given receptor subtype. In addition, in some GPCRs, where the orthosteric binding site is not clear or its structure is poorly defined, the allosteric binding site might be a good alternative to target with small molecules; this has been observed in receptors with long peptidic ligands and is frequently found with the class B GPCRs (which are GPCRs characterized of having a long N-terminal extracellular domain). In general, the advantages of allosteric modulators apply regardless of the specific therapeutic area or the tissue where the receptor is being targeted.

2.1 The challenge of agonist dependence

Radioligand binding and functional assays have particular advantages when they are used to screen for allosteric modulators of GPCRs. Nevertheless, the extent and direction (that is positive or negative) of the interaction between the allosteric and orthosteric ligand for receptors with more than one endogenous ligand will depend on the orthosteric agonist interacting with the receptor; this phenomenon is known as probe or agonist dependence (**Figure 1**). Agonist dependence makes more complex the identification and pharmacological characterization of allosteric modulators. Particularly, the case of aplaviroc (an allosteric modulator for CC-chemokine receptor 5) showed no effect in the binding of CCL5 to the receptor but totally prevented the binding of CCL3 [9].

Agonist dependence, or better known as probe dependence, can seriously affect potential therapeutics and also the development of allosteric ligands. In the ideal situation, the endogenous ligand would be used as a prototypic ligand in the high throughput screening process during drug development. However, in a real situation, the endogenous agonists, most of the time are unsuitable and susceptible to rapid degradation along the drug screening process and even more during *in vivo* studies. For this reason, highly stable agonists are preferentially used. Therefore, the allosteric ligand is first tested with the natural ligand on an early stage of the process in order to conclude if the achieved effects are equivalent to those registered with the prototypical agonist.

In order to better illustrate this concept a good example would be when a PAM has the ability to increase the cholinergic neuronal transmission in Alzheimer's disease [10], but the endogenous ligand acetylcholine is of rapid degradation making it unsuitable for drug screening. Cholinergic substitute ligands such as carbachol or pilocarpine are used for screening, and the stable analog oxotremorine is used to validate the effects of muscarinic acetylcholine receptor (mAChR) allosteric modulators *in vivo* [11]. However, the effects of the PAM LY2033298 are dependent on the orthosteric agonist (carbachol or pilocarpine) being used [12, 13] and these effects could lead to unexpected profiles of the allosteric ligand in later stages of the drug discovery process.

The characteristic of some allosteric ligands to have differential probe dependence on multiple receptor subtypes is an additional consideration that can have significant implications for the drug screening process. For instance, LY2033298 was reported to be a specific positive allosteric modulator of the M4 mAChR. Accordingly, PAM LY2033298 increased acetylcholine-mediated calcium responses at the M4 mAChR but not for the rest of the four receptor subtypes [14]. This allosteric modulator has also been shown to have high positive cooperativity with the surrogate orthosteric ligands oxotremorine and tetramethylammonium at the M2 mAChR [13]; this positive cooperative effect is similar to that observed with LY2033298 and oxotremorine at the M4 mAChR. This is an example of how the probe-dependent interaction of oxotremorine at both the M2 and M4 receptor subtypes can confound experimental interpretation of the effect of the allosteric ligand *in vivo* [11]. This highlights the need to understand the probe dependence of allosteric ligands at related receptors to ensure a robust target validation.

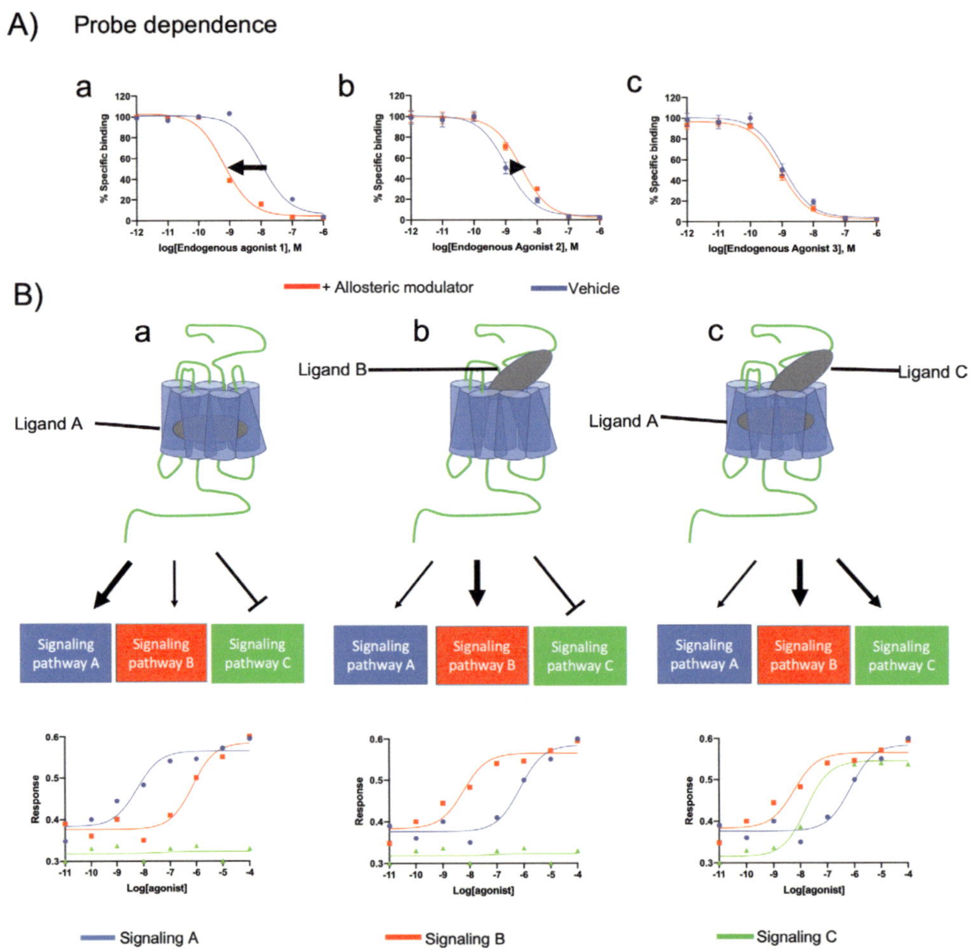

Figure 1.
Agonist dependence and biased agonism. (A) Agonist dependence of an allosteric ligand is shown with several endogenous agonists. (Aa) An allosteric modulator potentiates the ability of endogenous Agonist-1 to inhibit the binding of an antagonist to a human GPCR. (Ab) An allosteric modulator displaying weak or almost neutral cooperativity with endogenous Agonist-2. (Ac) An allosteric modulator displaying neutral cooperativity with endogenous Agonist-3. (B) Biased agonism is the capacity of different agonists to differentially activate the same GPCR, producing specific sets of signaling pathways. Changes in efficacy or potency by different agonists are indicators of potential biased agonism for a given GPCR. (Ba) Allosteric modulator-A showing stronger potency for signaling-A than for signaling-B, and not showing effect at signaling-C. (Bb) Allosteric modulator-B displaying higher potency for signaling-B than for signaling-A. (Bc) A biased agonist in complex with a GPCR can by itself preferentially activate to a unique set of signaling pathways and the interaction of the ligand-GPCR complex with an allosteric ligand will affect the signaling bias of the GPCR. Ligand-C is co-bound with an allosteric modulator-A and it potentiates the stimulus towards pathway-B and generates activity on signaling-C, however it down regulates signaling-A. This can be observed by a change in potency and efficacy between signaling-B and signaling-C in comparison with signaling-A.

Probe dependence is irrelevant in many physiological systems because the therapeutically targeted GPCRs have only one endogenous ligand. However, as we mentioned above, receptors can also respond to several endogenous agonists, under physiological conditions and disease. It is important to mention few more examples like the case of the chemokine receptors [15], melanocortin receptors [16], parathyroid hormone receptor 1 [17], relaxin receptors [18], calcium-sensing receptors [19], calcitonin and calcitonin-like receptors [20], as well as glucagon and glucagon-like peptide 1 (GLP1) receptors [21] and galanin receptors. In these examples, agonist dependence represents a huge challenge in the development of allosteric ligands as well as their therapeutic application.

2.2 Biased agonism in allosteric modulation

Distinct ligands can show different capacities to differentially activate signaling pathways from a GPCR by inducing different structural conformations [8, 22]; this effect is termed as biased signaling (also known as biased agonism see **Figure 2**). Examples of ligands that produce biased signaling include classical orthosteric adrenoceptor antagonists and inverse agonists (also known as beta-blockers) that antagonize receptor-mediated cyclic AMP production but promote cAMP response element-mediated gene transcription [23].

Research of carvedilol, an adrenoceptor antagonist, has shown to be a superior therapeutic, as compared to other adrenoceptor antagonists, for heart failure therapy [24] Despite that the drug was shown to be an inverse agonist for Gαs dependent signaling, it was also observed that carvedilol exerts partial agonism inβ -arrestin-dependent extracellular signal-regulated kinase 1 (ERK1) and ERK2 phosphorylation [25]. Based on these observations we can hypothesize that a different set of efficacies in different signaling pathways determines the final therapeutic outcome of GPCR ligands. Biased signaling has been widely studied for orthosteric ligands, however, there is also the possibility that many, if not all allosteric ligands, will exert biased signaling properties when the receptor is co-bound to the agonist.

At the present time, the terms biased agonism and allosteric modulation are usually considered to be different pharmacological phenomena. However, both events share in common that they are due to ligand-specific conformational changes in the GPCR that implicates a change in the three-dimensional structure of the GPCR. Having as a result that some specific signaling pathways can be either positively or negatively regulated.

For instance, the allosteric modulators of parturition (PDC113.824) induce biased signaling when an orthosteric ligand is co-bound to the prostaglandin F2α receptor. In mouse models, this compound acts as a negative allosteric modulator of prostaglandin F2α receptor-mediated cytosolic calcium oscillations and myometrial contraction. Specifically, PDC113.824 uncouples the receptor from the Gα12–RHO–ROCK (RHO-associated protein kinase) signaling pathway, but still significantly increases the phosphorylation of ERK1 and ERK2 Gαq dependent [26]. An auto-antibody for the calcium-sensing receptor that produces acquired hypocalciuric hypercalcemia by selectively increasing Gαq-dependent signaling and inhibiting

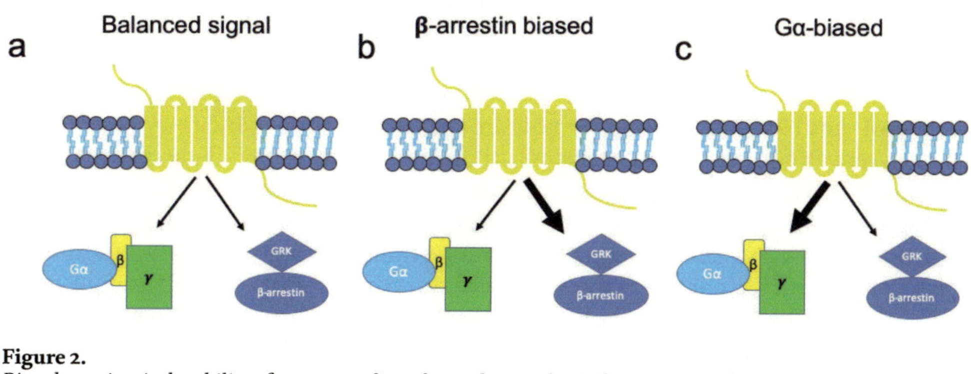

Figure 2.
Biased agonism is the ability of a receptor-ligand complex to selectively activate its downstream signaling pathways. (a) A balanced signal that stimulates both signaling pathways, G-protein dependent or β-arrestin dependent, equally in the same manner. (b) A biased ligand acting on the receptor as an agonist of one pathway (e.g., β-arrestins) while acting as an antagonist of another pathway (e.g., through heterotrimeric G proteins). (c) A biased ligand acting on the receptor as an agonist of one pathway (e.g., through heterotrimeric G proteins) while acting as an antagonist of another pathway (e.g., beta-arrestins).

Gαi-dependent signaling [27]. This is only one example of how an allosteric modulator can induce biased signaling that results in disease.

Based on these examples is that we can see the need to deeply understand the effect of allosteric modulation at different signaling pathways, as positive and negative regulation of every pathway from the receptor, does not always generate a beneficial therapeutic effect.

In theory, the operational model describes that biased agonism via allosteric modulation is a pathway-dependent variation in the signaling produced by the agonist in such a way that is not correlated with the intrinsic efficacy of the agonist or allosteric modulators [28]. However, in real conditions, biased signaling by an allosteric modulator is when the allosteric ligand potentiates one pathway but decreases the other one, as we previously described.

For a better understanding of this pharmacological phenomenon, we can continue describing more examples in this regard. Another very good example is the case of the allosteric modulation of the muscarinic receptor M4 subtype (M4 mAChR). Increasing signaling at M4 mAChR by the allosteric modulator LY2033298 generated significant changes in the grade of positive cooperativity in various signaling cascades of this receptor [29]. An additional case to exemplify this is the biased allosteric modulation of the GLP1 receptor. Some allosteric ligands can potentiate cAMP production and having a smaller effect on β-arrestin dependent signaling [30, 31].

Currently, most allosteric modulators have been discovered following screening assays; such as those used to identify agonists and antagonists, instead of a thoughtful rational process. The development of novel allosteric modulators that can induce biased agonism has the potential of specifically targeting therapeutic signaling pathways and excluding off-target pathways providing in this way a novel mechanism of biased agonism and produce new drugs with fewer side effects. However, we also face the problem that poses a big challenge in drug discovery and development of allosteric ligands and is that for the vast majority of GPCRs, it is still not well understood which set of signaling pathways efficacies will produce the desired therapeutic effect. The most important issue in the development of biased allosteric ligands is required a full understanding of the molecular determinants and also structural signatures that will lead to biased signaling on a receptor.

2.3 Agonist dependence in allosteric modulation and biased agonism

Many GPCRs have more than one endogenous agonist in such a way that their action is differentially regulated by the same allosteric modulator, having, as a result, a phenomenon called probe dependence. For instance, in the case of GLP1 receptor, there are two PAMs (compound 2 and BETP (4-(3-benzyloxyphenyl)-2-ethylsulfinyl-6-(trifluoromethyl) pyrimidine)) that show agonist dependence; where they increased the affinity of the oxyntomodulin (an endogenous agonist) by 18–25 times respectively. In contrast, none of them had no effect on four more ligands of GLP1 receptor [30, 32]. Interestingly, these allosteric modulators induced biased signaling during GLP-1 activation by oxyntomodulin. Observing an increase in Gαs activation, β-arrestin1/2 recruitment and insulin secretion, but they did not show any allosteric effect in ERK1/2 activation. The capacity of a modulator to regulate all or only some endogenous ligands in a pathway-dependent manner could not only seriously affect the development of novel allosteric modulators but also their therapeutics.

2.4 Implications in drug screening

Currently, allosteric screening routinely relies on seeking compounds that regulate the actions of the main endogenous ligand. Conversely, screening against alternative endogenous ligands, even if they have lower affinity or efficacy, may yield new leads that might not be possible to identify if screening for cooperative effects is only performed using the main endogenous ligand.

The possibility that an allosteric modulator will antagonize or potentiate the effects of an endogenous agonist without affecting other endogenous agonists would be seen as a therapeutic advantage, only in the case that each agonist exerts a different physiological effect. For example, according to previous studies some CCR5 allosteric modulators prevent the interaction of HIV-1 to CCR5, inhibiting in this way the infection [33]. However, it has not been well understood, whether inhibiting the chemokine physiological function of CCR5, would be desirable from a therapeutic point of view. During AIDS treatment, it is highly desirable the availability of allosteric modulators that prevent the HIV-1 entry without affecting CCR5 internalization by chemokines, since CCR5 plays a key role in favorable protection in the progression of AIDs after HIV-1 infection [34].

Probe dependent effects and the capacity of allosteric ligands to induce allosteric bias could be used to regulate GPCR physiological function in such a way that the signaling pathways that lead to favorable physiological outputs can be selectively targeted.

2.5 GPCR structure and allosteric modulation

All GPCRs are involved in nearly all physiological functions in humans and are the target of intense drug discovery efforts [35, 36]. Recent structures of GPCRs bound to allosteric modulators have revealed that the receptor surface is characterized by diverse cavities and crevices that may serve as binding sites for allosteric modulators [37]. This supports the notion that GPCRs are structurally flexible and they can be regulated by different allosteric ligands through a wide variety of mechanisms [38–43]. The vast majority of these structures have been solved with NAMs, which stabilize receptors in their inactive states [37]. Currently, only a single structure of an active GPCR bound to a small-molecule PAM has been described, the M2 muscarinic acetylcholine receptor with LY2119620 [44]. Thus, mechanisms of PAMs and their potential binding sites remain unexplored.

2.6 Therapeutic relevance

Receptor subtypes have orthosteric sites that are similar in its tridimensional structure and sometimes even in their amino acid sequence since mutations within this site, may especially decrease receptor function with detrimental consequences for the system. This can be harmful in complex systems and thus, evolution does not frequently favor such changes. In contrast, allosteric binding sites are less critical for receptor function and this is why they often have great structural variation between receptor subtypes. Moreover, in contrast to orthosteric ligands, allosteric drugs have the potential of being highly specific by only targeting a very specific set of receptor subtypes. But also, it is worth to highlight that the same allosteric site might be structurally different across species, having as a consequence differential effects of the same allosteric ligand between species [45].

Allosteric ligands cannot activate or inactivate receptors. Specifically, allosteric action will depend on endogenous ligands like neurotrophins, hormones, nucleotides or lipid moieties whose levels in the organism are tightly regulated. This can lower overdose risk relative to similarly acting orthosteric drugs. It may also allow a strategy where large enough doses that saturate all the receptors of the target tissue can be administrated to prolong the drug effect [5]. These characteristics enable receptors to be activated at specific times (i.e., in response to a physiological stimulus) with the difference of the constant activation by an orthosteric agonist [45].

Allosteric ligands regulate the responses already existing within tissues and making possible the drug response on specific tissue. Contrary to orthosteric ligands where they produce a less targeted effect within the organism since they bind to every receptor they can, affecting multiple tissues expressing the target receptor [1].

Some allosteric modulators have also been shown to lack the desensitizing effect that some agonists. Nicotinic acetylcholine receptors, for example, quickly desensitize in the presence of agonist drugs but maintain normal function in the presence of PAMs [46].

3. Conclusions

A huge number of drugs with fewer side effects are being developed using allosteric targets. Only two types of screening strategies are the principal approach in drug discovery; phage display and high-throughput screening. It is foreseen that complex computations will be conducted in years to come in order to gain better insights about the binding pockets within the receptors for which allosteric modulators can potentially be designed [47–49]. Information from crystal structures of receptors bound to different ligands would provide structural insights about the conformational changes that occur upon ligand binding. These studies would be fundamental during a rational drug design of these kind of ligands. In the last few years, we have seen a great advance in the design of novel allosteric modulators and it will possibly intensify even more in the near future. Progress in drug delivery will help to obtain further spatial specificity of therapeutic drugs, and as a result, we expect will translate into identifying significantly increased number of new drug possibilities that are more effective and with fewer side effects [50, 51]. However, no matter how selective such drugs can be designed, they cannot equalize the spatiotemporal basis of specificity that occurs naturally in our systems. Therefore, every single advance in allosteric drug discovery that promotes the homeostasis of our biological systems, will significantly contribute to the goals of developing more effective drugs with fewer side effects.

Acknowledgements

This work was supported by grants from the National Institute of Health, the American Heart Association, and Robert J. Kleberg, Jr. and Helen C. Kleberg Foundation.

Conflict of interest

The authors declare no conflict of interest.

Author details

Arfaxad Reyes-Alcaraz*, Emilio Y. Lucero Garcia-Rojas, Richard A. Bond and Bradley K. McConnell
College of Pharmacy, University of Houston, Houston, TX, USA

*Address all correspondence to: areyesa2@central.uh.edu

References

[1] Kenakin TP. Pharmacology in Drug Discovery and Development: Understanding Drug Response. Cambridge, MA: Academic Press; 2017. pp. 102-119

[2] Kenakin T, Strachan RT. PAM-antagonists: A better way to block pathological receptor signaling? Trends in Pharmacological Sciences. 2018;**39**(8):748-765

[3] Furchgott RF. Receptor mechanisms. Annual Review of Pharmacology. 1964;**4**:21-50

[4] Ariens EJ. Affinity and intrinsic activity in the theory of competitive inhibition. I. Problems and theory. Archives Internationales de Pharmacodynamie et de Thérapie. 1954. p. 32-49

[5] Rang HP, Ritter J, Flower R, Henderson G. Rang and Dale's Pharmacology. Amsterdam Netherlands: Elsevier; 2016. pp. 6-20

[6] Neubig RR, S. M, Kenakin T, Christopoulos A. International Union of Pharmacology Committee on receptor nomenclature and drug classification. XXXVIII. Update on terms and symbols in quantitative pharmacology. Pharmacological Reviews. 2003;**55**:597-606

[7] Jin R, Clark S, Weeks AM, Dudman JT, Gouaux E, Partin KM. Mechanism of positive allosteric modulators acting on AMPA receptors. The Journal of Neuroscience. 2005;**25**:9027-9036

[8] Kenakin T, Miller LJ. Seven transmembrane receptors as shapeshifting proteins: The impact of allosteric modulation and functional selectivity on new drug discovery. Pharmacological Reviews. 2010;**62**(2):265-304

[9] Watson C et al. The CCR5 receptor-based mechanism of action of 873140, a potent allosteric noncompetitive HIV entry inhibitor. Molecular Pharmacology. 2005;**67**(4):1268-1282

[10] Krause RM, Buisson B, Bertrand S, Corringer PJ, Galzi JL, Changeux JP, et al. Ivermectin: A positive allosteric effector of the α7 neuronal nicotinic acetylcholine receptor. Molecular Pharmacology. 1997;**53**:283-294

[11] Suratman S, Leach K, Sexton P, Felder C, Loiacono R, Christopoulos A. Impact of species variability and "probe-dependence" on the detection and in vivo validation of allosteric modulation at the M4 muscarinic acetylcholine receptor. British Journal of Pharmacology. 2010;**162**:1659-1670

[12] Vindhya Nawaratne KL, Christian C, Felder, Sexton PM, Christopoulos A. Structural determinants of allosteric agonism and modulation at the M4 muscarinic acetylcholine receptor identification of ligand-specific and global activation mechanisms. The Journal of Biiological Chemistry. 2010;**285**:19012-19021

[13] Valant C, J RL, Patrick M, Sexton, Christopoulos A. The best of both worlds? Bitopic orthosteric/allosteric ligands of G protein-coupled receptors. Annual Review of Pharmacology and Toxicology. 2012;**52**:153-178

[14] Chan WY, McKinzie DL, Bose S, Mitchell SN, Witkin JM, Thompson RC, et al. Allosteric modulation of the muscarinic M4 receptor as an approach to treating schizophrenia. Proceedings of the National Academy of Science. 2008;**105**:10978-10983

[15] Charo IF, Ransohoff RM. The many roles of chemokines and chemokine receptors in inflammation. The

New England Journal of Medicine. 2006;**354**:610-621

[16] Tao Y-X. The melanocortin-4 receptor: Physiology, pharmacology, and pathophysiology. Endocrine Reviews. 2010;**31**:506-543

[17] Gardella TJ, Jüppner H. Interaction of PTH and PTHrP with their receptors. Reviews in Endocrine & Metabolic Disorders. 2000;**1**:317-329

[18] Halls ML, van der Westhuizen ET, Bathgate RAD, Summers RJ. Relaxin family peptide receptors—Former orphans reunite with their parent ligands to activate multiple signalling pathways. British Journal of Pharmacology. 2007;**150**:677-691

[19] Conigrave AD, Quinn SJ, Brown EM. L-amino acid sensing by the extracellular Ca^{2+}-sensing receptor. Proceedings of the National Academy of Science. 2000;**97**:4814-4819

[20] Poyner DR, Sexton PM, Marshall I, Smith DM, Quirion R, Born W, et al. International Union of Pharmacology. XXXII. The mammalian calcitonin gene-related peptides, adrenomedullin, amylin, and calcitonin receptors. Pharmacological Reviews. 2002;**54**:233-246

[21] Estall JL, Drucker DJ. Glucagon and glucagon-like peptide receptors as drug targets. Current Pharmaceutical Design. 2006;**12**(14):1731-1750

[22] Katie Leach PMS, Christopoulos A. Allosteric GPCR modulators: Taking advantage of permissive receptor pharmacology. Trends in Pharmacological Sciences. 2007;**28**(8):382-389

[23] Baker JG, Hall IP, Hill SJ. Agonist and inverse agonist actions of β-blockers at the human β2-adrenoceptor provide evidence for agonist-directed signaling. Molecular Pharmacology. 2003;**64**:1357-1369

[24] Fröhlich H, Zhao J, Täger T, Cebola R, Schellberg D, Katus HA, et al. Carvedilol compared with metoprolol succinate in the treatment and prognosis of patients with stable chronic heart failure: Carvedilol or metoprolol evaluation study. Circulation Heart Failure. 2015;**8**:887-896

[25] Wisler JW, DeWire SM, Whalen EJ, Violin JD, Drake MM, Ahn S, et al. A unique mechanism of β-blocker action: Carvedilol stimulates β-arrestin signaling. Proceedings of the National Academy of Science. 2007;**104**:16657-16662

[26] Goupil E, Tassy D, Bourguet C, Quiniou C, Wisehart V, Pétrin D, et al. A novel biased allosteric compound inhibitor of parturition selectively impedes the prostaglandin F2α-mediated rho/ROCK signaling pathway. The Journal of Biological Chemistry, 2010;**285**:25624-25636

[27] Noriko Makita JS, Manaka K, Shoji Y, Oishi A, Hashimoto M, Fujita T, et al. An acquired hypocalciuric hypercalcemia autoantibody induces allosteric transition among active human Ca-sensing receptor conformations. Proceedings of the National Academy of Science. 2007;**104**:5443-5448

[28] Canals M, Sexton PM, Christopoulos A. Allostery in GPCRs: 'MWC' revisited. Trends in Biochemical Sciences. 2011;**36**(12):663-672

[29] Leach K, Loiacono RE, Felder CC, DL MK, Mogg A, Shaw DB, et al. Molecular mechanisms of action and In vivo validation of an M4 muscarinic acetylcholine receptor allosteric modulator with potential antipsychotic properties. Neuropsychopharmacology. 2010;**35**:855-869

[30] Koole C, Wootten D, Simms J, Valant C, Sridhar R, Woodman OL, et al. Allosteric ligands of the glucagon-like

peptide 1 receptor (GLP-1R) differentially modulate endogenous and exogenous peptide responses in a pathway-selective manner: Implications for drug screening. Molecular Pharmacology. 2010;**78**:456-465

[31] Wootten D, Savage EE, Valant C, May LT, Sloop KW, Ficorilli J, et al. Allosteric modulation of endogenous metabolites as an avenue for drug discovery. Molecular Pharmacology. 2012;**82**:281-290

[32] Willard FS, Wootten D, Showalter AD, Savage EE, Ficorilli J, Farb TB, et al. Small molecule allosteric modulation of the glucagon-like Peptide-1 receptor enhances the insulinotropic effect of oxyntomodulin. Molecular Pharmacology. 2012;**82**:1066-1073

[33] Muniz-Medina VM, Jones S, Maglich JM, Galardi C, Hollingsworth RE, Kazmierski WM, et al. The relative activity of "function sparing" HIV-1 entry inhibitors on viral entry and CCR5 internalization: Is allosteric functional selectivity a valuable therapeutic property? Molecular Pharmacology. 2009;**75**:490-501

[34] Gonzalez E, Kulkarni H, Bolivar H, Mangano A, Sanchez R, Catano G, et al. The influence of CCL3L1 gene-containing segmental duplications on HIV-1/AIDS susceptibility. Science. 2005;**307**:1434-1440

[35] Pierce KL, Premont RT, Lefkowitz RJ. Seven-transmembrane receptors. Nature Reviews Molecular Cell Biology. 2002;**3**:639-650

[36] Alexander S, Hauser MMA, Rask-Andersen M, Schiöth HB, Gloriam DE. Trends in GPCR drug discovery: New agents, targets and indications. Nature Reviews. Drug Discovery. 2017;**16**:829-842

[37] Thal DM, Glukhova A, Sexton PM, Christopoulos A. Structural insights into G-protein-coupled receptor allostery. Nature. 2018;**559**:45-53

[38] Wacker D, Stevens RC, Roth BL. How ligands illuminate GPCR molecular pharmacology. Cell. 2017;**170**:414-427

[39] Staus DP, Strachan RT, Manglik A, Pani B, Kahsai AW, Kim TH, et al. Allosteric nanobodies reveal the dynamic range and diverse mechanisms of G-protein-coupled receptor activation. Nature. 2016;**535**:448-452

[40] Manglik A, Kim TH, Masureel M, Altenbach C, Yang Z, Hilger D, et al. Structural insights into the dynamic process of β2-adrenergic receptor signaling. Cell;**161**:1001-1011

[41] Ye L, Van Eps N, Zimmer M, Ernst OP, Prosser RS. Activation of the A2A adenosine G-protein-coupled receptor by conformational selection. Nature. 2016;**533**:265-268

[42] Ned Van Eps LNC, Morizumi T, Kusnetzow AK, Szczepek M, Hofmann KP, Bayburt TH, et al. Conformational equilibria of light-activated rhodopsin in nanodiscs. Proceedings of the National Academy of Science. 2017;**114**:E3268-E3275

[43] Dror RO, Green HF, Valant C, Borhani DW, Valcourt JR, Pan AC, et al. Structural basis for modulation of a G-protein-coupled receptor by allosteric drugs. Nature. 2013;**503**:295-299

[44] Kruse AC, Ring AM, Manglik A, Hu J, Hu K, Eitel K, et al. Activation and allosteric modulation of a muscarinic acetylcholine receptor. Nature. 2013;**504**:101-106

[45] Lu S, He X, Ni D, Zhang J. Allosteric modulator discovery: From serendipity to structure-based design.

Journal of Medicinal Chemistry. 2019;**62**:6405-6421

[46] Williams DK, Wang J, Papke RL. Positive allosteric modulators as an approach to nicotinic acetylcholine receptor-targeted therapeutics: Advantages and limitations. Biochemical Pharmacology. 2011;**82**(8):915-930

[47] Wilhelm A, Lopez-Garcia LA, Busschots K, Fröhner W, Maurer F, Boettcher S, et al. 2-(3-Oxo-1,3-diphenylpropyl)malonic acids as potent allosteric ligands of the PIF pocket of phosphoinositide-dependent kinase-1: Development and prodrug concept. Journal of Medicinal Chemistry;**55**:9817-9830

[48] Hindie V, Lopez-Garcia LA, Biondi RM. Use of a fluorescent ATP analog to probe the allosteric conformational change in the active site of the protein kinase PDK1. Methods in Molecular Biology. 2012;**928**:133-141

[49] Laine E, Martínez L, Ladant D, Malliavin T, Blondel A. Molecular motions as a drug target: Mechanistic simulations of anthrax toxin edema factor function led to the discovery of novel allosteric inhibitors. Toxins (Basel). 2012;**4**:580-604

[50] Kalia Y, Perozzo R, Scapozza L. The pharmaceutical biochemistry group: Where pharmaceutical chemistry meets biology and drug delivery. Chimia (Aarau). 2012;**66**:313-319

[51] Allémann E, Delie F, Lange N. Pharmaceutical technology at the service of targeted drug delivery. Chimia (Aarau). 2012;**66**:308-312

Chapter 6

Potassium Channels as a Potential Target Spot for Drugs

Vladimir Djokic and Radmila Novakovic

Abstract

Aberrant function or expression of potassium channels can be underlying in pathologies such as cardiac arrhythmia, diabetes mellitus, hypertension, preterm birth, and various types of cancer. The expression of potassium channels is altered in many types of diseases. Also, we have previously shown that natural polyphenols, such as resveratrol, and selective synthetic modulators of potassium channels, like pinacidil, can alter their function and lead to the desired outcome. Therefore, targeting potassium channels with substance, which has an influence on their function, is promising access to cancer, diabetes mellitus, preterm birth, or hypertension therapy. In this chapter, we could discuss strategies for targeting different types of potassium channels as potential targets for synthetic and natural molecules therapy.

Keywords: potassium channels, K channels, modulators of K channels, activators, inhibitors, natural polyphenols, resveratrol, K channels antibody

1. Introduction

Ion channels are protein molecules that form pores in the cell membrane and membranes of cellular organelles and allow passive flow of ions in the direction of their electrochemical gradient and result in electrical currents. Ion channels play key roles in membrane potential generation and many cellular activities such as signal transduction, neurotransmitter release, muscle contraction, hormone secretion, volume regulation, growth, motility, and apoptosis [1].

It is widely known that potassium channels (K channels) are transmembrane proteins that allow the flow of potassium across the membrane to regulate ion homeostasis, cell proliferation, migration, cell volume, and specific processes such as muscular contraction [2].

K channels are the most diverse ion channel type, and each subtype has a specific physiological role. K channels are highly attractive as targets for the development of novel therapeutics. However, the lack of detailed structural and functional insight of K channels and their diversity and ubiquity pose challenges for the development of selective drug candidates.

For many years the structure and types of K channels were unknown due to the lack of specific ligands for their activation or blocking. A progressive shift in the study of these structures has emerged since the discovery of animal toxins that are highly specific to individual types but also with the introduction of electrophysiological methods—voltage clamp and patch clamp, which have made it possible to test individual channel. In recent years, many genes detected participate in the encoding of these ion channels. Some subtypes are cloned and their biophysical properties determined, but this has not led to a complete elucidation of their function [3]. Especially in recent years, studies on this membrane protein family in different tissue types dramatically increased. Parallel with this remarkable progress in our understanding of molecular diversity, structure, and function, a growing number of discoveries have linked K channel gene mutations with various diseases. Such diseases of the heart, kidney, pancreas, and central nervous system involve either mutation(s) in the K channel gene(s) and/or altered regulation of K channel function. The enhanced understanding of these diseases, facilitated by a combination of genomic and biophysical approaches, has helped our understanding of how various mutations affect channel function, contribute to disease etiology, and rationalize novel treatment strategies.

This review will survey the K channels crucial role in the physiologic and pathophysiological function and discuss the emerging understanding of their clinical influence. Once taken into account these strategies, K channels may represent suitable and easily accessible different disease biomarkers and targets for therapy.

2. Classification of K channels

Ion channels classified according to the type of ions they conduct, their structure, their expression pattern and mode of activation [4]. Potassium channels are composed of complexes of several protein subunits, each encoded by a different gene.

The general model of the K channel is a complex of four α subunits grouped in the form of a pore through the membrane. Two transmembrane helices and a short loop between them (called the P-loop) are trademarks of these channels. The P-loop contains the amino acid sequence of threonine-valine-glycine-tyrosine-glycine, which is the selective filter most responsible for the selective passage of K^+ ions through the channel. This architecture with two transmembrane helices and a loop is an essential and universal feature of the K channel, but further, different features characterize each channel subfamily. In addition to α subunits, a variety of accessory-regulatory subunits such as SUR, β, MinK, and KChiP and others enter the K channel composition [5].

Different types of K channels have been shown to comprise more than 100 different protein subunits that are tissue-specific and species-specific [6]. About 75 genes coding different types of K channels have detected in human genomes. Molecular studies of K channels have allowed their classification based on the primary amino acid sequence of the pore-containing subunit. This sequence motif, conserved across all K channels, was proposed to correspond to the selectivity filter of the pore-forming region of the channel protein. There are many (sub)types and isoforms of K channels divided into three groups based on transmembrane domains that make up the α subunit [3]. These channels are classified into three groups, based on the number of transmembrane domains (TMDs) (**Figure 1**). Within each family, ion channels with 65% identical amino acid sequences are further grouped into subfamilies [7]. The standard nomenclature for K channels is proposed by the *International Union of Basic and Clinical Pharmacology Committee on Receptor Nomenclature and Drug Classification* (NC-IUPHAR) [8], presented in **Figure 1** and **Tables 1–4**.

Orange is a Kv type with six transmembrane domains, with red main subtypes K_{Ca} channels; green is a Kir subtype with four transmembrane domains, and blue is a subtype with two transmembrane domains K_{2P}.

Understanding the role of K channels and detecting their subunits/proteins in different physiological and pathophysiological condition are essential, along with linking dysfunction of these channels to specific diseases and disorders. These facts speak to the importance of these channels, as a possible therapeutic site for the action of drugs that should prevent or stop unwanted conditions/states. Therefore, the study of their function and the expression of their proteins are of great importance.

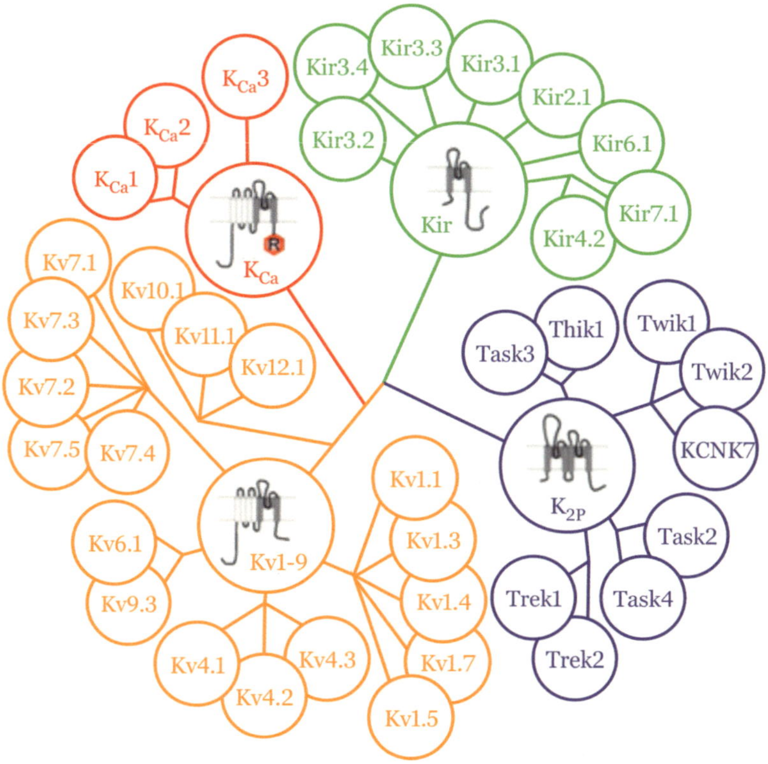

Figure 1.
Classification of main types and subtypes of K channels.

2.1 Voltage-dependent K channels (Kv) and their modulators

Kv channels are the largest superfamily of the K channel, coding with about 40 genes and containing 12 subfamilies, each with several representatives [9]. Representatives of Kv1–4, 7, and 10–12 subfamilies can form functional channels as homomers, while Kv5, 6, 8, and 9 must associate with Kv2 or three subunits to form a functional channel. The official nomenclature for Kv channels is Kva.b, where a and b denote the subfamily and ordinal number of channel discovery (**Figure 1**). There are six transmembrane domains in each subunit, designated as S1–S6. Four β-subunits are associated with α-subunits and located on the cytoplasmic side of the membrane [10]. There is a peptide loop between the S5 and S6 domains. Loops of α-subunits face the lumen of the pores and contribute to the formation of K^+ conductive pores [3]. Domain S4 is the central part of the voltage sensor necessary to activate the Kv channel. The opening/closing mechanism also contributes to the electrostatic interaction of negative charges on the S2 and S3 domains [11].

The biophysical properties, physiological regulation, and pharmacological properties of Kv channels are dependent on the combination of α subunits. The combination on four α subunits may be homo- or heteromultimers. Even more complex to these heteromultimers is their interaction with smaller accessory proteins including β subunits, KChIP, KchAP, and minK proteins, miRP peptide, and others [12, 13].

The isoforms of Kv channels dominant for smooth muscle are mainly Kv1, Kv2, Kv3, and Kv4. For example, in vascular smooth muscle cells, the most important subtypes of Kv channels are Kv1 (Kv1.1, Kv1.2, Kv1.3, Kv1.5, Kv1.6), Kv2 (Kv2.1), Kv3 (Kv3.1). Kv4 (Kv4 .2–3), and Kv7 (Kv7.1–5); in the smooth muscle of the uterus is Kv4 (Kv4.2, Kv4.3).

Activators	Inhibitors	Subtypes	Heteromultimers
-	α-dendrotoxin, margatoxin, tetraethylammonium (TEA)	Kv1.1	K_v1.2, K_v1.4, $K_v\beta$1 i $K_v\beta$2
-	margatoxin, α-dendrotoxin, noksiustoxin	Kv1.2	K_v1.1, K_v1.4, K_v β1 i K_v β2
-	margatoxin, noxiustoxin, TEA, maurotoxin, correolide	Kv1.3	K_v1.1, K_v1.2, K_v1.4, K_v1.6, K_v β1 i K_v β2
-	fampridine	Kv1.4	K_v1.1, K_v1.2, $K_v\beta$1 i $K_v\beta$2
-	fampridine	Kv1.5	$K_v\beta$1 i $K_v\beta$2
-	α-dendrotoxin, TEA	Kv1.6	$K_v\beta$1 i $K_v\beta$2
-	noxiustoxin, fampridine	Kv1.7	$K_v\beta$1 i $K_v\beta$2
-	fampridine	Kv1.8	$K_v\beta$1 i $K_v\beta$2
-	TEA	Kv2.1	K_v5.1, K_v6.1-6.4, K_v8.1-8.2, K_v9.1-9.3
-	fampridine, TEA	Kv2.2	K_v5.1, K_v6.1-6.4, K_v8.1-8.2, K_v9.1-9.3
-	fampridine, TEA	Kv3.1	-
-	fampridine, TEA	Kv3.2	-
-	TEA	Kv3.3	-
-	TEA	Kv3.4	MiRP2
-	fampridine	Kv4.1	KChIP 1-4, DP66, DPP10
-	-	Kv4.2	KChIP 1-4, DPP6, DPP10, $K_v\beta$1, NCS-1, Navβ1
-	-	Kv4.3	KChIP 1-4, DPP6 and DPP10, MinK, MiRPs
-	-	Kv5.1	-
-	-	Kv6.1	-
-	-	Kv6.2	-

-	-	Kv6.3	-
-	-	Kv6.4	-
-	XE991, linopiridine	Kv7.1	-
retigabine	XE991, linopiridine, TEA	Kv7.2	-
gabapentin, retigabine	linopiridine	Kv7.3	-
retigabine	XE991, linopiridine, TEA	Kv7.4	-
retigabine, gabapentin	linopiridine, XE991	Kv7.5	-
-	-	Kv8.1	-
-	-	Kv8.2	-
-	-	Kv9.1	-
-	-	Kv9.2	-
-	-	Kv9.3	-
-	LY97241, terfenadine, dofetilide, kalmodulin, astemizole	Kv10.1	-
-	LY97241, hinidin	Kv10.2	-
RPR260243	astemizole, terfenadin, disopyramide, E4031, dofetilide, ibutilide	Kv11.1	minK, MiRP1
-	E4031	Kv11.2	minK
-	E4031	Kv11.3	minK
-	Ba^{2+}	Kv12.1	minK
-	Cs^{+}	Kv12.2	minK, MiRP1

Table 1.
Selective modulators of voltage-sensitive channels.

The expression pattern depends on the compartment and/or conditions like gravid or not in the uterus and part of lent blood vessels. This heteromultimerization seems to modulate Kv current expression, sensitivity to various substances, as well as biophysical properties of channels such as inactivation [14–18]. Further, research shows that the most important isoforms for the proliferation, activation, migration, and apoptosis of tumor cells are Kv1.3, Kv1.5, Kv2.1, Kv41, Kv9.3, Kv10.1, and Kv11.1 [19].

A recognizable feature of Kv channels is their sensitivity to pharmacological modulators. The compounds most commonly used to inhibit Kv channels are 4-aminopyridine (4-AP) and tetraethylammonium (TEA). In general, Kv channels of vascular smooth muscle cells exhibit higher sensitivity to 4-AP, which nonspecifically inhibits members of the Kv1–4 subfamilies of these channels [20]. Electrophysiological imaging showed that the channels encoded by Kv1.2 and Kv1.5 genes were relatively sensitive to 4-AP, while Kv2 channels inhibited TEA more effectively. The 4-AP concentrations required for the half-maximal inhibition of Kv channel function varied between 0.3 mM and 1.1 mM. These differences in channel sensitivity attribute to the different expressions of Kv channel subtypes, the use of different animal species in studies, differences in sex, cell isolation techniques, and imaging conditions [12, 20].

2.1.1 *Ca^{2+}- and voltage-dependent K channels (KCa) channels and their modulators*

Ca^{2+}-sensitive Kv channels other than voltage-dependent depolarizations, for opening, also require an increased concentration of Ca^{2+} ions in the cytoplasm [21]. They are divided into channels with high ($K_{Ca}1$-BK_{Ca}, maxi K, 100–300 pS), intermediate ($K_{Ca}3$-IK_{Ca}, 25–100 pS), and low conductivity ($K_{Ca}2$-SK_{Ca}, 2–25 pS) [22]. $K_{Ca}1$ channels are activated by membrane depolarization and/or Ca^{2+} binding to the channel; $K_{Ca}2$ and $K_{Ca}3$ channels are voltage-independent and activated by Ca^{2+} binding to calmodulin that constitutively binds to the channels [23].

$K_{Ca}1.1$ channels form of α pore-forming subunits and auxiliary β or γ subunits. The four α subunits can build a functional channel on their own. Associated accessory subunits act as potent regulators of most channel characteristics, including voltage and Ca^{2+} sensitivity, as well as sensitivity to pharmacological modulators.

The differences in $K_{Ca}1.1$ channels and Kv channels are the presence of an additional transmembrane (S0) segment with the extracellular N-terminus, as well as the presence of a long intracellular C-terminus, forming the so-called "channel tail." Furthermore, unlike Kv channels, where the voltage sensor is localizing in the S4 domain, the positively charged residues responsible for the voltage dependence of the $K_{Ca}1.1$ channels are less centralized and present in the S2, S3, and S4 domains [21]. There are different intracellular partners of these channels. Also, $K_{Ca}1.1$ channels can be the targets of a number of posttranslational modifications such as oxidation, glycosylation, and phosphorylation reactions. Finally, the association of α subunits with different regulatory subunits further contributes to increasing the diversity of these channels [23, 24].

Furthermore, four types of β subunits (β1–4) and four types of γ subunits (γ1–4) modulate almost all the physiological and pharmacological properties of

Activators	Inhibitors	Subtypes
NS004, NS1619	paxilline, caribdotoxin , iberiotoxin, TEA	$K_{Ca}1.1$
EBIO, NS309	apamin, UCL1684, TEA	$K_{Ca}2.1$
NS309, EBIO	UCL1684, apamin, TEA	$K_{Ca}2.2$
EBIO, NS309	apamin, UCL1684, TEA	$K_{Ca}2.3$
NS309, EBIO SKA-121	caribdotoxin, TRAM-34, senikapok	$K_{Ca}3.1$

Table 2.
Selective modulators of Ca^{2+}- and voltage-sensitive channels (K_{Ca}).

$K_{Ca}1.1$ channels. β subunits contain two, while γ subunits are constructed from a single transmembrane domain. The mechanism by which helper subunits interact with α subunits and regulate $K_{Ca}1.1$ channel activity is extremely complicated, but it is critical for the study and understanding of the vascular disease. In vascular smooth muscle cells, the β1 subunit is the predominant isoform, and its dysfunction is associated with diabetes, hypertension, and other vascular diseases. Deletion of the gene for the β1 subunit causes a significant decrease in Ca^{2+}-sensitivity of the channel. As auxiliary subunits of $K_{Ca}1.1$ channels, γ subunits also affect their activity by modulating voltage and Ca^{2+}-dependence. They play a role in the regulation of smooth muscle tone, and change in the gene encoding them leads to a decrease in the activity of functional $K_{Ca}1.1$ channels lead to constrictions [25–27]. Expression of β1 subunit can be selectively upstream or downstream-regulated in smooth muscle cells, without reflecting to α subunit expression. Occurs under the influence of various physiological and pathophysiological conditions, as well as during hormonal stimulation and that increase or decrease the channel activity [26, 28].

$K_{Ca}1.1$ channels also represent important targets in the mechanism of action of various activators or inhibitors. Adenosine and β-adrenergic agonists activate $K_{Ca}1.1$ channels via cAMP-dependent and cGMP-dependent pathways. Especially in vascular smooth muscle cells, elevated levels of cGMP and activation of PKG with NO result in the phosphorylation of BKCa and their subsequent activation. On the other hand, angiotensin II and endothelin-1 inhibit $K_{Ca}1.1$ channels in coronary arteries by PKC-independent mechanisms [29].

The pharmacology of $K_{Ca}1.1$ channels spread from nonspecific blockade with TEA and alkaloids, like paxillin, to more effective specific inhibitors scorpion toxins, such as iberiotoxin and charybdotoxin. Although these compounds do not have pure therapeutic potential, they are very useful tools for studying the function of these channels. Several small-molecule $K_{Ca}1.1$ channel openers have been detected for both native and cloned channels. For example, benzimidazole NS-1619 activates $K_{Ca}1.1$ channels, but its functional effects also include inhibition of Ca^{2+} currents and Kv channels. And many other substances can modulate the activity of $K_{Ca}1.1$ channels, such as estrogen, reactive oxygen species and ethanol [22, 30, 31].

$K_{Ca}2.1$, $K_{Ca}2.2$, and $K_{Ca}3.1$ channels are mostly present in neurons, endothelium of the blood vessels, epithelium, and in several types of smooth muscle, e.g., in the urinary tract. Thus, the opening of these channels is independent of the membrane potential but strictly dependent on Ca^{2+}. Complex Ca^{2+} calmodulin induces a conformational change leading to the opening of the pore [32].

Pharmacologically, $K_{Ca}2$ channels are highly sensitive to bee venom and apamin with different affinity for all channel isoforms: $K_{Ca}2$ channels are the most sensitive and $K_{Ca}1$ the least. Scilatoxin, biculculin, dequalinium, and its more potent derivative UCL1684 are also potent inhibitors of these channels group. The compounds, such as clotrimazole and TRAM-34, are more specific inhibitors of $K_{Ca}3.1$ channel. $K_{Ca}3.1$ current can be reduced by the scorpion toxin charybdotoxin, like $K_{Ca}1.1$ channels. Both types of channels are activated by chlorzoxazone, zoxazolamine, riluzole, 1-EBIO, its more potent DC-EBIO derivative, and NS-309. However, these compounds are not successful, such as Ca^{2+} for channel activation. Moreover, an increase in channel sensitivity for Ca^{2+} is an assumed mechanism of their action [31].

2.2 Inwardly rectifying K channels (Kir) and their modulators

The inwardly rectifying (Kir) channels conduct K^+ ions into the cell at a membrane potential more negative than the equilibrium potential for K^+, while at more positive potentials, the output K^+ current is limited and barely detectable [33]. The explanation for the phenomenon of inward rectification is in the fact that intracellular Mg^{2+} and polyamines (spermine and spermidine) block output K^+ currents.

As carriers of positive charge, polyamines and Mg^{2+} interact with the negatively charged amino acids present in the transmembrane M1 domain and terminal C-terminus of the Kir channel, thereby inhibiting the passage of K^+ ions through the pore [34]. Kir channels have been identified in many types of cells. Seven subfamilies are identified so far (**Figure 1** and **Table 3**).

Structure of Kir channel is consisting of four α subunit-forming subunits, each containing two transmembrane domains (M1 and M2) and a P-loop between them. The properties and functions of Kir channels vary between different tissues and species. For example, Kir channel expression is most pronounced in the smooth muscle of the autoregulatory vascular compartments, such as the coronary and cerebral circulation. Kir duct expression increases with decreased blood vessel diameter. The difference in expressive Kir channels can be explained by the fact that the conduction artery shows a very small response to a smaller version of extracellular K, whereas resistant arteries show a positive response [35].

Activators	Inhibitors	Subtypes	Associated subunits
-	tertiapin-Q , Ba^{2+}, Cs^+	Kir1.1	-
PIP_2	spermine, spermidine, putrescine, Mg^{2+}, Ba^{2+}, Cs^+	Kir2.1	-
-	Mg^{2+}, Ba^{2+}, Cs^+	Kir2.2	-
-	Mg^{2+}, spermine, spermidine, putrescine, Ba^{2+}, Cs^+	Kir2.3	-
Mg^{2+}	Cs^+, Ba^{2+}	Kir2.4	-
PIP_2	tertiapin-Q , Ba^{2+}	Kir3.1	-
PIP_2	pimozide, desipramine	Kir3.2	-
PIP_2	-	Kir3.3	-
PIP_2	tertiapin-Q	Kir3.4	-
-	Ba^{2+}, Cs^+	Kir4.1	-
-	Ba^{2+}, Cs^+	Kir4.2	-
-	Ba^{2+}	Kir5.1	-
diazoxide,minoxidil nicorandil,cromakalim, pinacidil, resveratrol,	glibenclamide, tolbutamide	Kir6.1	SUR1, SUR2A, SUR2B
diazoxide,minoxidil nicorandil,cromakalim, pinacidil, resveratrol,	glibenclamide, tolbutamide	Kir6.2	SUR1, SUR2A, SUR2B
-	Ba^{2+}, Cs^+	Kir7.1	-

Table 3.
Selective modulators of inwardly rectifying K channels (Kir).

ATP-sensitive Kir channels (K_{ATP}) are the exceptions, which have a more complex heterooctamer structure with multiple types of accessory subunits [3, 5]. Structurally, K_{ATP} channels form of four pore-forming Kir6.x subunits and four regulatory subunits known as sulfonylurea receptors, SURx. Kir6.x subunits are responsible for ATP inhibition and SURx for nucleoside-diphosphate activation.

Functional expression of the K_{ATP} channel requires coexpression of Kir6.x and SURx subunits in a 1:1 ratio. SUR1 is predominantly present in pancreatic β cells. SUR2 has two variants, SUR2A and SUR2B, which are generated by alternative excision of exon 38 in the ABCC9 gene. SUR2A is mainly present in the myocardium and skeletal muscle, while SUR2B generally is distributed in the vascular and myometrial smooth muscle cells [17, 25, 35, 36].

Numerous studies have highlighted that K_{ATP} channels in vascular smooth muscle cells play an important role in achieving systemic vasodilation during hypoxia, increasing blood flow to the heart, kidney, and muscle. This vasodilation is attributed to the release of NO or adenosine due to hypoxia but also to the direct effect of hypoxia itself. During hypoxia, K_{ATP} channels may be activated by a decrease in ATP, a decrease in pH and partial pressure of oxygen, or an increase in intracellular lactates and ADP. These factors can activate K_{ATP} channels directly and/or potentiate NO activation [37].

K_{ATP} channels play their roles in the mechanism of the action of relaxation and contraction by interacting with various protein kinases. Thus, K_{ATP} channels activated by protein kinase A (PKA) and cGMP-dependent protein kinase participate in the mechanism of action of endogenous vasodilators such as adenosine and prostacyclin. On the other hand, activation of protein kinase C (PKC) and vasoconstrictor induced increases in intracellular Ca^{2+} caused by noradrenaline, vasopressin, endothelin, and angiotensin II were accompanied by inhibition of the K_{ATP} channel [38–40].

K_{ATP} channels in the smooth muscle are inhibited by antidiabetics from a group of sulfonylurea derivatives, such as glibenclamide and tolbutamide. Glibenclamide is the most commonly used K_{ATP} channel inhibitor in vascular smooth muscle studies, whereas tolbutamide shows much lower potency [13, 41].

In the study of potential drugs, the core interest is directed towards K_{ATP} channels, since they exhibit activity under basic conditions and significantly contribute to the control of the resting membrane potential [42].

2.3 K channels with two pores (K_{2P}) and their modulators

K_{2P} channel subunit consists of two regions that participate in pore formation (P1 and P2, hence their name) and four transmembrane domains (M1–M4). Functional channels form as dimers of these subunits that form a single pore selectively permeable to potassium [43]. Activity of these channels is voltage-independent, and they under physiological conditions (high concentration of K^+ in the cytoplasm and low extracellular) conduct K^+ ions from the cell into the extracellular space [44], leading to stability of the resting membrane potential. K_{2P} channel activity is regulated by a wide variety of factors such as pH, stretching of membrane, temperature, and endogenic compounds like arachidonic acid. K_{2P} channels play important roles in many physiological processes: neuroprotection, cerebrovascular vasodilation, regulation of aldosterone production and secretion, depression, chemoreception, and pulmonary vasoconstriction [45].

The neuroprotective agent riluzole, currently in use for the treatment of amyotrophic lateral sclerosis, has been shown to be an activator of TREK-1 and TRAAK channels. Volatile general anesthetics such as chloroform and isoflurane have also been shown to target TREK-1 channels [3].

Activators	Inhibitors	Subtypes
-	-	$K_{2P}1.1$/TWIK1
arachidonic acid, halothane, chloroform, isoflurane, membrane elongation, heat, acidic pH	norfluoxetine	$K_{2P}2.1$/TREK1
halothane	methanandamide, anandamide, acidic pH	$K_{2P}3.1$/TASK1
arachidonic acid, riluzole, membrane elongation, heat	-	$K_{2P}4.1$/TRAAK
-	-	$K_{2P}5.1$/TASK2
-	-	$K_{2P}6.1$/TWIK2
-	-	$K_{2P}7.1$
halothane	methanandamide, anandamide	$K_{2P}9.1$/TASK3
arachidonic acid, halothane, membrane elongation	-	$K_{2P}10.1$/TREK2
-	-	$K_{2P}12.1$/THIK2
-	halothane	$K_{2P}13.1$/THIK1
-	-	$K_{2P}15.1$/TASK5
acidic pH	-	$K_{2P}16.1$/TALK1
acidic pH	-	$K_{2P}17.1$/TALK2
-	arachidonic acid	$K_{2P}18.1$/TRESK

Table 4.
Selective modulators of K channels with two pores K_{2P}

3. Natural polyphenols and antibody for K channels a promise for future cancer treatment

3.1 Natural polyphenols

Natural polyphenols are secondary metabolism of plants that have multiple activities in determining plant properties such as color, aroma, taste, solution, pathogen resistance, etc. Natural polyphenols have been expanding in the interest of both the scientific community and the public over the past decade when they have shown to have a significant function in the prevention of cancer, cardiovascular disease, diabetes and neurodegenerative disorders, etc. [46–49]. Polyphenols are the most common antioxidant constituents, and their source is various foods of plant origin: fruits, vegetables, seeds, especially nuts, chocolate, wine, tea, and coffee.

Research carried out during the last decade provided evidence that natural, biologically active polyphenols, such as resveratrol, genistein, quercetin, and catechin-gallate, and curcumin have a wide spectrum of pharmacologic properties such as anti-inflammatory, antioxidant, anticarcinogenic, antiaging, neuroprotective, and cardioprotective effect. Resveratrol, stilbene from grape and red wine, genistein, isoflavone from soy-based food, and catechin-gallate from tea influence cancer initiation, promotion, and progression through diverse signal-transduction pathways that control cell growth and division, inflammation, apoptosis, metastasis, and angiogenesis [50].

Many studies suggested that Kv channels could be the targets of polyphenols, directly and indirectly [17, 47, 51]. Furthermore, there is evidence that modulation of Kv channels via the PI_3K/Akt/mTOR pathway may be a possible indirect mode of action of polyphenols [52, 53]. The PI_3K/Akt/mTOR pathway is known to play an important role in cell survival (inhibition of apoptosis), proliferation, and cell metabolism, and PI_3K activity has been linked to a variety of human cancers [54]. As described above, the effect on the kinase pathway would result in the modulation of K channel function.

Polyphenols are thought to have several different mechanisms that prevent cardiovascular disease. The following effects are reported in the literature: antioxidant, anti-aggregation, beneficial effects on plasma HDL-cholesterol levels (raising HDL-cholesterol levels), inhibition of LDL-cholesterol oxidation, improvement of endothelial function, and stabilization of atherosclerotic plaque [55]. The mechanism of the vasodilatory action of polyphenols is not fully understood. Still, there are many results that polyphenols included K channels in their mechanism of action [46–48]. It is shown that these molecules can cause endothelium-dependent and endothelium-independent relaxation of the blood vessel. Polyphenols are known to modulate many intracellular signaling pathways as well as the expression of individual genes. Thus, plant polyphenols have been described to activate endothelial NO synthase (eNOS), increase nitric oxide production, and thus induce endothelium-dependent vasodilation. Activation of eNOS occurs due to an increase in the intracellular level of Ca^{2+} ions and phosphorylation of PI_3 kinase.

Previous reports indicated that resveratrol inhibits vasocontractile response and relaxes different arteries and vein by the activation of smooth muscle Kv and $K_{Ca}1.1$ channels [47, 48]. But, data from electrophysiological studies suggest that resveratrol inhibits L-type Ca^{2+} channels and enhances activity of the K_{ATP} channels in rat hearts [51].

Additionally, it has been shown that the K channel family affects cell function and plays a significant role in regulating myometrium contractility [5, 19]. Changes in the expression or activity of K channels can translate into inadequate repolarization leading to aberrant uterine activity. Thus, K channel alterations may contribute to certain pathophysiological conditions such as preterm labor. Many studies have shown that opening of different types of K channels leads to the relaxation of nonpregnant as well as pregnant myometrium [5, 17, 19, 26, 56]. It seems that function and molecular expression of K channels are dependent of stages of pregnancy, the age, and of hormones influences [17, 57]. K channels, as a novel target to prevent preterm delivery with nontoxic natural polyphenols, are the important work in addressing the need for innovative tocolytic therapeutics.

In such a scenario, combination treatment with K channel modulators and natural polyphenols could be beneficial for cardiovascular, renal, or gynecologic disorders.

3.2 Antibodies

The increasing knowledge on the expression of K channels in tumors, together with the information on the structure and function of these molecules and the possibility of detailed in vitro and in vivo studies, makes this family of channels an attractive candidate for the design of personalized therapies for oncological diseases.

As already stated, in addition to regulating many physiological functions, K channels are aberrantly expressed in different types of tumors. In cancer cells, K channel activity regulates cell proliferation, resistance to apoptotic cell death, tumor angiogenesis, invasiveness, and metastatic spread. Moreover, being expressed in cells of the tumor microenvironment, K channels can also modulate the immune/inflammatory response, which contributes to the drive of cancer establishment and progression [18, 58]. After many years of studies, some K channels are emerging as novel cancer biomarkers, to be employed to stratify patients for either prognostic or predictive purposes [59].

Although the attempts to generate blocking monoclonal antibodies using conventional approaches have shown limited success, the insight that structural studies have provided in the last few years makes it possible to design alternative strategies with higher chances of success. This opens doors for a new approach to combine the advantageous features of K channels-specific antibodies and their modulators and will undoubtedly result in improved therapy alternatives in the near future.

It anticipates that a detailed understanding of structural aspects would revolutionize and refine approaches targeting K channels for therapeutic purposes.

4. Conclusion

K channels are crucial for all aspects of life by regulating the excitability of neurons and the heart, contracting muscles, secreting hormones, moving fluid, and activating the immune cell. K channel modulation accordingly offers tremendous opportunities for drug development. However, with 7% of clinically used drugs targeting ligand-ion channels and only 5% of voltage-gated channels targeted, ion channels are currently "underrepresented" drugs in clinical practice [60]. The reason for this discrepancy is the fact that K channels belonging to a single subtype can be found in the different tissues, e.g., the heart and brain, where they play different roles in the nervous excitability and contractility of the heart muscle. It was mentioned above that even within the same tissue there are subtypes of channels that potentially play different roles in disease and physiology, thus making sub-selective modulators of each subtype of K channels desirable as candidates for drug development. The ubiquity of K channels makes it important to develop highly selective agents. Furthermore, numerous studies have shown that different diseases as diabetes mellitus and hypertension cause changes in K channel expression and function that further complicate solution innovative sub-selective therapeutics or antibodies. However, it is not remote the time in which it will be possible to target specific K channels for therapeutic purposes.

Conflict of interest

The author declares no conflict of interest.

Funding

This work was supported by the Scientific Research Grant from Ministry of Education, Science, and Technological Development Government of the Republic of Serbia [No TR31020, OI175064].

Author details

Vladimir Djokic and Radmila Novakovic*
Faculty of Medicine, Institute of Pharmacology, Clinical Pharmacology and Toxicology, University of Belgrade, Belgrade, Serbia

*Address all correspondence to: radmila.novakovic@med.bg.ac.rs

References

[1] Kim JB. Channelopathies. Korean Journal of Pediatrics. 2014;**57**:1-18

[2] Ashcroft FM. Ion Channels and Disease. Academic Press; 2000

[3] Shieh CC, Coghlan M, Sullivan JP, Gopalakrishnan M. Potassium channels: Molecular defects, diseases, and therapeutic opportunities. Pharmacological Reviews. 2000;**52**(4):557-594

[4] Shad KF, Salman S, Afridi S, Tariq M, Asghar S. Introductory chapter; Ion channels. In: Shad KF, editor. Ion Channels in Health and Sickness. Rijeka: IntechOpen; 2018. DOI: 10.5772/intechopen.72025. ISBN: 978-1-78984-228-9

[5] Khan RN, Matharoo-Ball B, Arulkumaran S, Ashford ML. Potassium channels in the human myometrium. Experimental Physiology. 2001;**86**:255-264

[6] Miller C. An overview of the potassium channel family. Genome Biology. 2000;**1**(4):0004.1-0004.5. Available from: http://genomebiology.com/2000/1/4/reviews/0004

[7] Jenkinson DH. Potassium channels—Multiplicity and challenges. British Journal of Pharmacology. 2006;**147**:63-71

[8] Alexander SPH, Mathie A, Peters JA, Veale EL, Striessnig J, Kelly E, et al. The concise guide to pharmacology 2019/20: Ion channels. British Journal of Pharmacology 2019:142-228

[9] Monsuez JJ. Cardiac potassium currents and channels—Part I: Basic science aspects. International Journal of Cardiology. 1997;**61**(3):209-219

[10] Seoh SA, Sigg D, Papazian DM, Bezanilla F. Voltage-sensing residues in the S2 and S4 segments of the Shaker K+ channel. Neuron. 1996;**16**(6):1159-1167

[11] Joseph BK, Thakali KM, Moore CL, Rhee SW. Ion channel remodeling in vascular smooth muscle during hypertension: Implications for novel therapeutic approaches. Pharmacological Research. 2013;**70**(1):126-138

[12] Ko EA, Park WS, Firth AL, Kim N, Yuan JX, Han J. Patophysiology of voltage gated K+ channels in vascular smooth muscle cells: Modulation by protein kinases. Progress in Biophysics and Molecular Biology. 2010;**103**:95-101

[13] Castle NA. Pharmacological modulation of voltage-gated potassium channels as a therapeutic strategy. Expert Opinion on Therapeutic Patents. 2010;**20**(11):1471-1503

[14] Werner EM, Ledoux J. K+ channels in biological processes: Vascular K+ channels in the regulation of blood pressure. Journal of Receptor, Ligand and Channel Research. 2014;**7**:51-60

[15] Nieves-Cintrón M, Syed AU, Buonarati OR, Rigor RR, Nystoriak MA, Ghosh D, et al. Impaired BKCa channel function in native vascular smooth muscle from humans with type 2 diabetes. Scientific Reports. 2017;**7**:14058

[16] Smith RC, McClure MC, Smith MA, Abel PW, Bradley ME. The role of voltage-gated potassium channels in the regulation of mouse uterine contractility. Reproductive Biology and Endocrinology. 2007;**5**:41

[17] Novakovic R, Radunovic N, Markovic-Lipkovski J, Cirovic S, Beleslin-Cokic B, Ilic B, et al. Effects of the polyphenol resveratrol on contractility of human term pregnant

myometrium. Molecular Human Reproduction. 2015;**21**(6):545-551

[18] Hernandez-Resendiz I, Hartung F, Pardo LA. Antibodies targeting KV potassium channels: A promising treatment for cancer. Bioelectricity;**1**(3):180-187

[19] Brainard AM, Korovkina VP, England SK. Potassium channels and uterine function. Seminars in Cell & Developmental Biology. 2007;**18**:332-339

[20] Jackson WF. KV channels and the regulation of vascular smooth muscle tone. Microcirculation. 2018;**25**:e12421

[21] Tykocki NR, Boerman EM, Jackson WF. Smooth muscle ion channels and regulation of vascular tone in resistance arteries and arterioles. Comprehensive Physiology. 2017;7(2):485-581

[22] Carvalho de Souza JL, Varanda WA, Tostes RC, Chignalia AZ. BK channels in cardiovascular diseases and aging. Aging and Disease. 2013;**4**(1):38-49

[23] Wei AD, Gutman GA, Aldrich R, Chandy KG, Grissmer S, Wulff H. International Union of Pharmacology. LII Nomenclature and molecular relationships of calcium-activated potassium channels. Pharmacological Reviews. 2005;**57**:463-472

[24] Lee US, Shi J, Cui J. Modulation of BK channel gating by the 2 subunit involves both membrane-spanning and cytoplasmic domains of Slo1. The Journal of Neuroscience. 2010;**30**:16170-16179

[25] Nimigean CM, Magleby KL. The β subunit increases the Ca^{2+} sensitivity of large conductance Ca^{2+}-activated potassium channels by retaining the gating in the bursting states. The Journal of General Physiology. 2002;**113**:425-440

[26] Novakovic R, Ilic B, Beleslin-Cokic B, Radunovic N, Heinle H, Scepanovic R, et al. The effect of resveratrol on contractility of non-pregnant rat uterus: The contribution of K(+) channels. Journal of Physiology and Pharmacology. 2013;**64**:795-805

[27] Zhu Y, Ye P, Chen SL, Zhang DM. Functional regulation of large conductance Ca2+-activated K+ channels in vascular diseases. Metabolism: Clinical and Experimental. 2018;**83**:75-80

[28] Amberg GC, Santana LF. Downregulation of the BK channel β1 subunit in genetic hypertension. Circulation Research. 2003;**93**:965-971

[29] Hu XQ, Zhang L. Function and regulation of large conductance Ca(2+)-activated K+ channel in vascular smooth muscle cells. Drug Discovery Today. 2012;**17**:974-987

[30] Gribkoff VK, Starrett JE Jr, Dworetzky SI. The pharmacology and molecular biology of large conductance calcium-activated (BK) potassium channels. Advances in Pharmacology. 1997;**37**:319-348

[31] Ledoux J, Werner ME, Brayden JE, Nelson MT. Calcium-activated potassium channels and the regulation of vascular tone. Physiology (Bethesda). 2006;**21**:69-78

[32] Dopico AM. Ethanol sensitivity of BK(Ca) channels from arterial smooth muscle does not require the presence of the beta 1-subunit. American Journal of Physiology. Cell Physiology. 2003;**284**:C1468-C1480

[33] Feletou M. Calcium-activated potassium channels and endothelial dysfunction: Therapeutic options? British Journal of Pharmacology. 2009;**156**:545-562

[34] Hille B. Ion Channels of Excitable Membranes. Sunderland, MA: Sinauer Associates, Inc; 2001

[35] Hibino H, Inanobe A, Furutani K, Murakami S, Findlay I, Kurachi Y. Inwardly rectifying potassium channels: Their structure, function, and physiological roles. Physiological Reviews. 2010;**90**(1):291-366

[36] Chrissobolis S, Sobey CG. Inwardly rectifying potassium channels in the regulation of vascular tone. Current Drug Targets. 2003;**4**(4):281-289

[37] Djokic V, Jankovic-Raznatovic S, Novakovic R, Kostic M, Rajkovic J, Labudovic-Borovic M, et al. Effect of gestational diabetes mellitus and pregnancy-induced hypertension on human umbilical vein smooth muscle KATP channels. Experimental and Molecular Pathology. 2019;**111**:104323. DOI: 10.1016/j.yexmp.2019.104323

[38] Landry DW, Oliver JA. The ATP-sensitive K+ channel mediates hypotension in endotoxemia and hypoxic lactic acidosis in dog. The Journal of Clinical Investigation. 1992;**89**:2071-2074

[39] Jackson WF. Potassium channels in the peripheral microcirculation. Microcirculation. 2005;**12**:113-127

[40] Ko EA, Han J, Jung ID, Park WS. Physiological roles of K+ channels in vascular smooth muscle cells. Journal of Smooth Muscle Research. 2008;**44**:65-81. DOI: 10.1540/jsmr.44.65

[41] Aguilar-Bryan L, Nichols CG, Wechsler SW, Clement JP 4th, Boyd AE 3rd, González G, et al. Cloning of the beta cell high-affinity sulfonylurea receptor: A regulator of insulin secretion. Science. 1995;**268**(5209):423-426

[42] Teramoto N. Physiological roles of ATP-sensitive K+ channels in smooth muscle. The Journal of Physiology. 2006;**572**(3):617-624

[43] Mathie A, Al-Moubarak E, Veale EL. Gating of two pore domain potassium channels. The Journal of Physiology. 2010;**588**(17):3149-3156

[44] Enyedi P, Czirjak G. Molecular background of leak K+ currents: Two-pore domain potassium channels. Physiological Reviews. 2010;**90**(2):559-605

[45] Gurney A, Manoury B. Two-pore potassium channels in the cardiovascular system. European Biophysics Journal. 2009;**38**(3):305-318

[46] Protić D, Beleslin-Čokić B, Novaković R, Kanjuh V, Heinle H, Sćepanović R, et al. Effect of wine polyphenol resveratrol on the contractions elicited electrically or by norepinephrine in the rat portal vein. Phytotherapy Research. 2013;**27**:1685-1693

[47] Gojkovic-Bukarica L, Markovic-Lipkovski J, Heinle H, Cirovic S, Rajkovic J, Djokic V, et al. The red wine polyphenol resveratrol induced relaxation of the isolated renal artery of diabetic rats: The role of potassium channels. Journal of Functional Foods. 2019;**52**:266-275

[48] Gojkovic Bukarica LJ, Protic D, Kanjuh V, Heinle H, Novakovic R, Šcepanovic R. Cardiovascular effects of resveratrol. Vojnosanitetski Pregled. 2013;**70**(12):1145-1150

[49] Scalbert A, Manach C, Morand C, Rémésy C, Jiménez L. Dietary polyphenols and the prevention of diseases. Critical Reviews in Food Science and Nutrition. 2005;**45**(4):287-306

[50] Afaq F, Katiyar SK. Polyphenols: Skin photoprotection and inhibition of photocarcinogenesis. Mini Reviews in Medicinal Chemistry. 2011;**11**(14):1200-1215

[51] Chen WP, Chi TC, Chuang LM, Su MJ. Resveratrol enhances insulin

secretion by blocking K (ATP) and K (V) channels of beta cells. European Journal of Pharmacology. 2007;**568**:269-277

[52] Kim YA, Kim GY, Park KY, Choi YH. Resveratrol inhibits nitric oxide and prostaglandin E2 production by lipopolysaccharide-activated C6 microglia. Journal of Medicinal Food. 2007;**10**(2):218-224

[53] Ko EA, Park WS, Son YK, Kim Do H, Kim N, Kim HK, et al. The effect of tyrosine kinase inhibitor genistein on voltage-dependent K+ channels in rabbit coronary arterial smooth muscle cells. Vascular Pharmacology. 2009;**50**:51-56

[54] Chamcheu JC, Roy T, Uddin MB, Banang-Mbeumi S, Chamcheu RN, Walker AL, Liu YY, Huang S. Role and therapeutic targeting of the PI3K/Akt/mTOR signaling pathway in skin cancer: A review of current status and future trends on natural and synthetic agents therapy. Cells. 2019;**8**(8). pii: E803. DOI: 10.3390/cells8080803

[55] Pandey KB, Rizvi SI. Plant polyphenols as dietary antioxidants in human health and disease. Oxidative Medicine and Cellular Longevity. 2009;**2**:270-278

[56] Novakovic R, Milovanovic S, Protic D, Djokic J, Heinle H, Gojkovic-Bukarica L. The effect of potassium channel opener pinacidil on the non-pregnant rat uterus. Basic & Clinical Pharmacology & Toxicology. 2007;**101**:181-186

[57] Lovasz N, Ducza E, Gaspar R, Falkay G. Ontogeny of sulfonylurea-binding regulatory subunits of KATP channels in the pregnant rat myometrium. Reproduction. 2011;**142**(1):175-181. DOI: 10.1530/rep-10-0492

[58] Pardo LA, Stuhmer W. The roles of K(+) channels in cancer. Nature Reviews. Cancer. 2013;**14**(1):39-48

[59] Cázares-Ordoñez V, Pardo LA. Kv10.1 potassium channel: From the brain to the tumors. Biochemistry and Cell Biology. 2017;**95**(5):531-536. DOI: 10.1139/bcb-2017-0062

[60] Gerlach AC, Antonio BM. Validation of ion channel targets. Channels (Austin, Tex.). 2015;**9**(6):376-379. DOI: 10.1080/19336950.2015.1081725

Chapter 7

Fibril Formation by Glucagon in Solution and in Membrane Environments

Akira Naito

Abstract

Glucagon is a 29-amino acid peptide hormone secreted by pancreatic α-cells and interacts with specific receptors located in various organs. Glucagon tends to form gel-like fibril aggregates that are cytotoxic because they activate apoptotic signaling pathways. First, fibril formation by glucagon in acidic solution is discussed in light of morphological and structural changes during elapsed time. Second, we provide kinetic analyses using a two-step autocatalytic reaction mechanism; the first step is a homogeneous nuclear formation process, and the second step is an autocatalytic heterogeneous fibril elongation process. Third, the processes of fibril formation by glucagon in a membrane environment are discussed based on the structural changes in the fibrils. In the presence of bicelles in acidic solution, glucagon interacts with the bicelles and forms fibril intermediates on the bicelle surface and grows into elongated fibrils. Glucagon-dimyristoylphosphatidylcholine (DMPC) bilayers in neutral solution mimic the environment for fibril formation by glucagon under near-physiological condition. Under these conditions, glucagon forms fibril intermediates that grow into elongated fibrils inside the lipid bilayer. Many days after preparing the glucagon-DMPC bilayer sample, the fibrils form networks inside and outside the bilayer. Furthermore, fibril intermediates strongly interact with lipid bilayers to form small particles.

Keywords: glucagon fibril, fibrillation mechanism, two-step autocatalytic reaction, lipid bilayer, solid-state NMR

1. Introduction

Glucagon is a 29-amino acid peptide hormone secreted by pancreatic α-cells and interacts with specific receptors located in various organs, where it activates the glycogenolysis and gluconeogenic pathways, resulting in raised blood glucose levels [1–3]. Glucagon tends to form gel-like fibrillar aggregates in acidic condition [4]. These aggregates are cytotoxic due to the activation of apoptotic signaling pathways [5]. These fibrils are similar to those of other therapeutic peptides and proteins such as human calcitonin (hCT) [6] and insulin [7] and pathologically related fibrils such as prion [8], amylin (type 2 diabetes) [9], β-amyloid (Alzheimer's disease) [10], and polyglutamine [11].

Some non-fibrillar proteins and peptides have been observed by electron microscopy to form amyloid fibrils with similar morphologies [12].

Several characteristics of these fibrils are related to the misfolding of proteins, leading to severe conditions such as fibril deposits in the brains of Alzheimer's disease patients [13] and in the pancreas of patients with type 2 diabetes [9].

Kinetic analyses of fibril formation by the therapeutic peptide human calcitonin indicate that hCT molecules associate to form fibril intermediates via a two-step autocatalytic reaction mechanism. The first step of kinetic reaction (rate constant, k_1) is a homogeneous reaction from micelle-like oligomers to fibril intermediates. These intermediates react with monomeric molecules to elongate into longer fibrils via a heterogeneous fibril elongation process (rate constant, k_2) [14–17]. Elucidating the molecular structure of amyloid fibrils is important for understanding the mechanism of self-aggregation, but it is difficult to determine high-resolution molecular structures using typical spectroscopic methods because fibrils are heterogeneous solids. Solid-state NMR spectroscopy has demonstrated advantages for the conformational determination of Alzheimer's amyloid β-peptides (Aβ), which mainly comprise 40 or 42 amino acid residues and are the main component of the amyloid plaques found in Alzheimer's disease patients [12, 18]. Both the intra-chain conformation of the Aβ molecule in fibrils and their intermolecular alignment have been analyzed to explore the mechanism of molecular association underlying the formation of Aβ (1–40) [19–21] and the more toxic Aβ (1–42) [22–24] fibrils.

The primary structure of the glucagon peptide is His^1-Ser-Gln-Gly-Thr^5-Phe-Thr-Ser-Asp-Tyr^{10}-Ser-Lys-Tyr-Leu-Asp^{15}-Ser-Arg-Arg-Ala-Gln^{20}-Asp-Phe-Val-Gln-Trp^{25}-Leu-Met-Asn-Thr-OH.

An X-ray crystallographic study showed that glucagon adopts a trimeric α-helix structure stabilized by hydrophobic interactions between molecules related by threefold symmetry [25], whereas a solution NMR study showed that glucagon in dilute aqueous solution may not form a specific structure, with the exception of the 22–25 region [26]. The secondary structure of glucagon in the presence of dodecylphosphocholine micelles comprises three turns of an irregular α-helix formed by residues 17 to 29 near the C-terminus, a stretch of extended polypeptide chain from residues 14 to 17, an α-helix-like turn formed by residue 10 to 14, and another extended region from residue 5 to 10 [27].

Fibril formation by glucagon molecules was observed by Beaven et al. in undisturbed aqueous solution at pH 2 [4]. The viscosity initially increased and a birefringent gel is formed. With time, a precipitate appeared comprising long fibrils, as determined using electron microscopy. Infrared spectra of the gel, solid film, and precipitate showed that in all these states, glucagon is in the form of antiparallel β-sheet chains [5, 28]. Kinetic analysis of fibril formation by glucagon under acidic conditions demonstrated a complex fibrillation mechanism in which suitable changes in the fibrillation condition can alter the type of fibril formed or result in the formation of a mixture of several types of fibrils [29, 30]. Furthermore, the fibrils come in two forms: one composed entirely of glucagon monomers and the other entirely of glucagon trimers [31]. Studies of fibril formation typically use acidic pH solutions because of the low solubility of glucagon in neutral solution.

Understanding the cytotoxicity of amyloid-forming peptides requires investigating the interaction of these peptides with membranes because lipid bilayer components dramatically alter most aspects of amyloid aggregation [32–35]. We previously reported glucagon fibrillation in the presence of dimyristoylphosphatidylcholine/1,2-dihexanoyl-sn-glycero-3-phophocholine (DMPC-DHPC) bicelles in acidic solution. The glucagon structure in the fibril in the presence of these bicelles is different from that in their absence [36]: the N- and C-termini both change from α-helix to β-sheet in acidic solution, while the N-terminus remains in an α-helical conformation, whereas the C-terminus changes from α-helix to β-sheet in the presence of bicelles. The nucleation rate is slower, and the fibril elongation rate is faster in acidic solution than in the presence of bicelles.

In neutral conditions, glucagon molecules are incorporated into lipid bilayers above the phase transition temperature, and the properties of the lipids appear to remain unperturbed. Below the phase transition temperature, glucagon forms discoidal particle with DMPC [37, 38] and induces closer packing of the phospholipid bilayers [39]. Similar peptide-lipid interaction to form discoidal particles below the phase transition temperature is seen in the melittin-DMPC bilayer system [40, 41].

The time course behavior of glucagon fibril formation inside a DMPC bilayer under neutral conditions, which approximates the physiological condition, and the kinetic behavior of glucagon under these conditions have been investigated to understand the fibrillation process under near-physiological conditions [42].

2. Fibril formation by glucagon in acidic solution

Gel formation by glucagon in the β-sheet conformation in acid solutions is a relatively slow process at room temperature [4] and can be followed by observing the change in viscosity as shown in **Figure 1**. The most marked feature of the change in viscosity in these time profiles is the presence of a substantial lag phase during which oligomeric nuclei are likely formed and function as initiation sites. These phenomena were confirmed by adding a small seed of preformed glucagon gel on the end of a wire into a viscometer containing a fresh acidic glucagon solution. The viscosity increased immediately with essentially no lag (**Figure 1a**). After a prolonged reaction time, the viscosity began to decrease and fibrils sometimes precipitated. These fibrils represent a variant of the β-structure of glucagon.

Fibril formation strongly depends on the peptide concentration, proceeding very slowly at less than about 1.5 mg/ml and occurring more readily at higher concentration (**Figure 1b**). Increasing the ionic strength of the solution results in both an increasing aggregation rate and more rapid production of fibrils. The change in viscosity with time in even 0.01 M sodium chloride occurs much more rapidly than in the absence of salt, and viscosity decreases quickly.

The effect of temperature on the polymerization rate is also very marked. Both the aggregation rate and the size of the aggregates as reflected in the maximal values of the reduced viscosity show a strong temperature maximum around 30°C (**Figure 1c**). An addition of 5% (v/v) of the nonaqueous solvent dioxin completely inhibits the aggregation (**Figure 1a**).

Transmission electron microscopy (TEM) time-elapsed pictures were obtained during fibril formation by glucagon dissolved in 0.015 M acetic acid solution (18 mg/ml) at pH 3.3 [36]. TEM pictures were measured approximately 2 hrs, then 1 week, and 6 months after the dissolution of glucagon (**Figure 2**). A small number of spherical-shaped fibril intermediates appeared after approximately 2 hrs, as shown in **Figure 2a**. After 1 week, the number of spherical fibril intermediates had increased, and elongated fibrils had appeared (**Figure 2b**). After 6 months, long mature fibrils about 10 nm in diameter were observed, and the spherical fibril intermediates had completely disappeared (**Figure 2c**).

The α-helical content of aged glucagon at 5.0 mg/ml decreased significantly to approximately 1%. The CD spectrum of a β-sheet structure typically shows an intense positive band at 198 nm and a negative band at 218 nm [5]. The CD spectral pattern of aged glucagon was that of a β-sheet structure, indicating a conformational transition from α-helical to β-sheet structure under these conditions.

The FTIR spectrum of glucagon immediately after dissolution showed a low-intensity β-sheet band at 1620–1630 cm^{-1}, and aging resulted in progressively

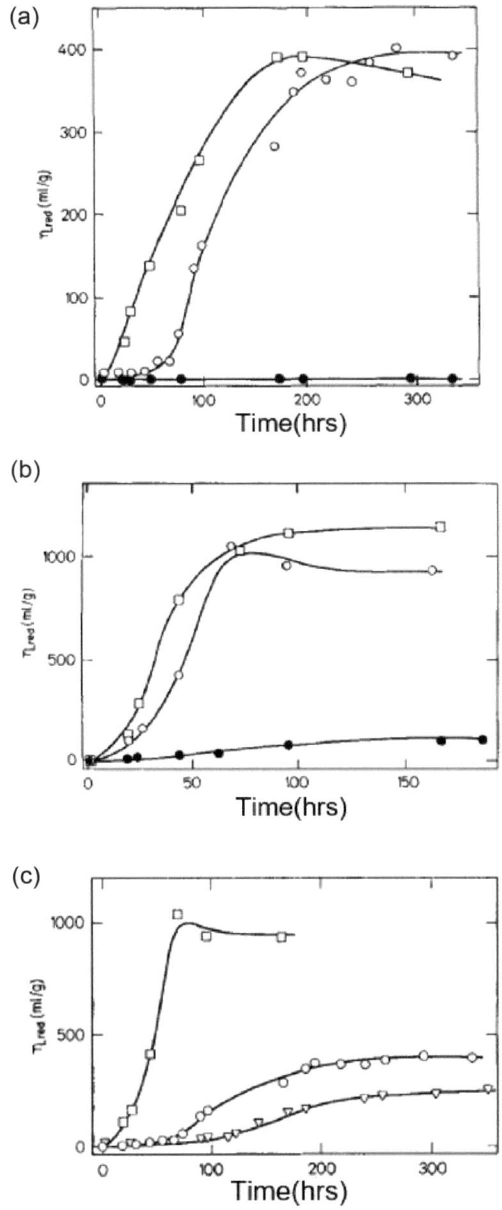

Figure 1.
Time course behavior of glucagon aggregation in 0.01 M hydrochloric acid at 26°C and a glucagon concentration of 2.5 mg/ml. (a) Time course of reduced viscosity (msp/c); glucagon with no addition (○); glucagon seeded with preformed gel (□); glucagon solution containing 5% by volume dioxin (●). (b) Effect of glucagon concentration at 4 mg/ml (□); 2.5 mg/ml (○); and 1 mg/ml (●). (c) Effect of temperature on the aggregation rate of glucagon at a glucagon concentration of 2.5 mg/ml at 26°C (○); 30°C (□); and 35°C (∇) (ref. [4]).

greater amounts of β-sheet [28]. Deconvolution and curve fitting of the amide I band showed that unaged glucagon contained 54% α-helix/random coil structure and 2% β-sheet structure, whereas aged glucagon comprised 22% α-helix/random coil structure and 49% β-sheet structure.

Detailed kinetic, spectroscopic, and morphological studies have revealed that glucagon can form several types of fibrils that differ at the level of molecular packing of the peptide [29–31, 43–46]. Each type forms through distinct nucleation-dependent aggregation pathways influenced by the solution conditions and can be self-propagated by seeding. Type A fibrils that form at high glucagon concentration (>5 mg/ml, pH 2.5) represent the least stable fibril type with a low melting midpoint (T_{mapp} < 32°C) and single protofilament fibrils observable by TEM (**Figure 3a**). Type B ($B_{unagitated}$ and $B_{agitated}$) fibrils form under low glucagon concentration (<0.5 mg/ml, pH 2.5). Type $B_{unagitated}$ fibrils grow by branching in the absence of agitation and appear as branched twisted fibrils by TEM (**Figure 3b**). Type $B_{agitated}$ glucagon fibrils form when the solution is agitated, suggesting that agitation breaks the fibril creating more free fibril ends that align as parallel pairs (**Figure 3c**). Type D fibrils grow under low glucagon concentration (<0.5 mg/ml, pH 2.5) in the presence of 150–250 mM Cl^- and are twisted and tightly packed

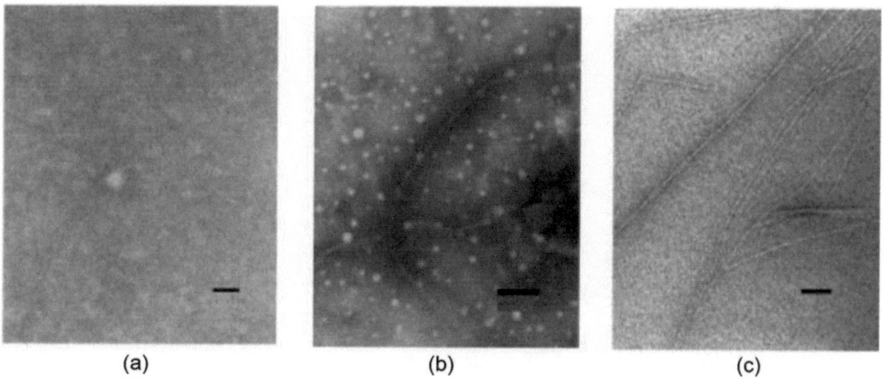

Figure 2.
Transmission electron micrographs of glucagon (18 mg/ml) in 0.015 M acetic acid solution at pH 3.3. (a) Taken approximately 2 hrs after the dissolution of glucagon. The bar indicates 20 nm. (b) Taken 1 week after dissolution of glucagon. The bar indicates 50 nm. (c) Taken 6 months after dissolution of glucagon. The bar indicates 50 nm (ref. [36]).

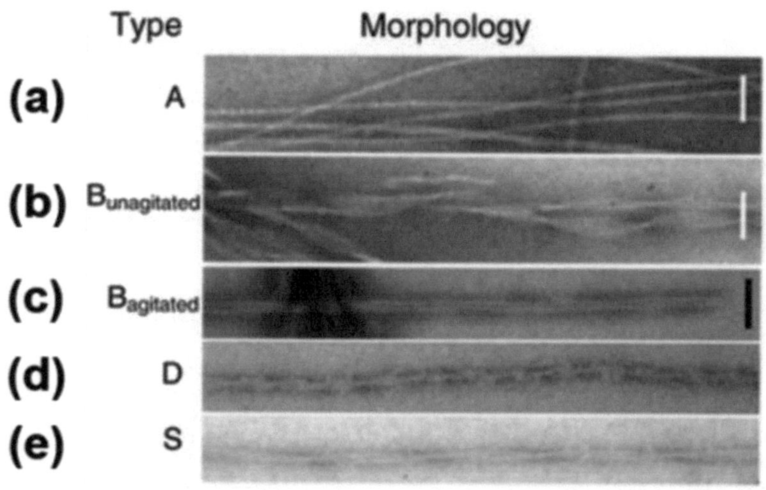

Figure 3.
Electron microscope image of morphology of different types of glucagon fibrils. The scale bar is 50 nm. (a) Type A: The glucagon concentration, >5 mg/ml, 50 mM glycine, pH 2.5, low agitation. (b) Type $B_{unagitated}$: Glucagon concentration, <0.5 mg/ml, 50 mM glycine, pH 2.5, low agitation. (c) Type $B_{agitated}$: Glucagon concentration, <0.5 mg/ml, 50 mM glycine, vigorous agitation. (d) Type D: Glucagon concentration, <0.5 mg/ml, 50 mM glycine, pH 2.5+, 150–250 mM Cl^-. (e) Type S: Glucagon concentration, <0.5 mg/ml, 0.01 N HCl, 1 mM SO_4^{2-} (ref. [30]).

(**Figure 3d**). Type S fibrils grow under low glucagon concentration (<0.5 mg/ml, pH 2.5) in the presence of 1 mM Na_2SO_4 (7:1 ratio with glucagon) and appear as twisted mature fibrils by TEM (**Figure 3e**).

Solid-state ^{13}C NMR spectra were observed for 18 mg/ml [1-^{13}C]Gly4 and [3-^{13}C]Ala19-glucagon in 0.015 M acetic acid solution, pH 3.3 [36]. The ^{13}C direct excitation with dipolar decoupling and magic angle spinning (DD-MAS) signal indicates monomeric glucagon, and the ^{13}C cross polarization with magic angle spinning (CP-MAS) signal indicates fibril glucagon. The DD-MAS spectra (**Figure 4A** and **C**) of [1-^{13}C]Gly4 and [3-^{13}C]Ala19 exhibit signals at 171.7 and 16.4 ppm, respectively, consistent with the monomeric state and indicate that the region near the Gly4 and Ala19 residues forms α-helix structures, as shown by the conformationally dependent chemical shift values [47–49]. The experimentally determined chemical shift values and secondary structures are summarized in **Table 1**. The ^{13}C CP-MAS spectra of [1-^{13}C]Gly4 and [3-^{13}C]Ala19 (**Figure 4B** and **D**)

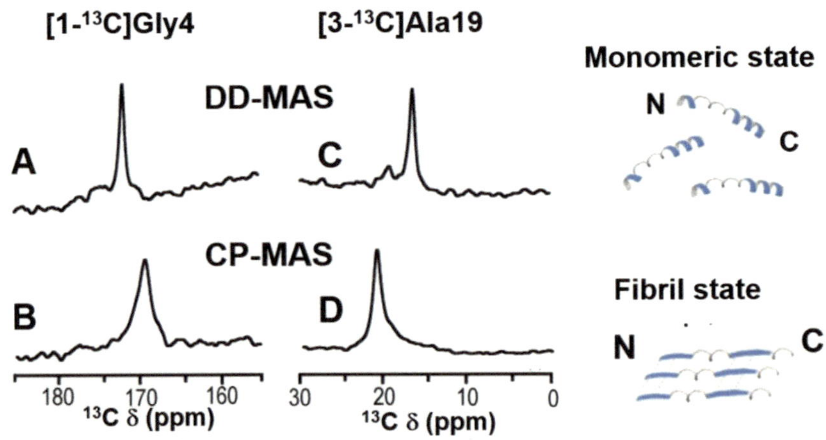

Figure 4.
^{13}C DD-MAS and CP-MAS NMR spectra of [1-^{13}C]Gly4 (A and B) and [3-^{13}C]Ala19 (C and D) of [1-^{13}C]Gly4 and [3-^{13}C]Ala19-glucagon in acetic acid solution at pH 3.3. Schematic structures of glucagon in the monomeric and fibril states (right panels) (ref. [36]).

Fibril formation condition	Fibril type	[1-^{13}C]Gly4 (structure)	[3-^{13}C]Ala19 (structure)	Ref.
Acidic solution (0.015 M acetic acid solution pH 3.3)	Monomer	171.7 (α-helix)	16.4 (α-helix)	[36]
	Fibril	169.2 (β-sheet)	21.0 (β-sheet)	[36]
Acidic solution in the presence of bicelle (DMPC+DHPC pH 3.3)	Monomer	171.5 (α-helix)	16.4 (α-sheet)	[36]
	Fibril	171.5 (α-helix)	19.3 (β-sheet)	[36]
Glucagon inside lipid bilayer (DMPC) in neutral solution	Monomer	171.5 (α-helix)	15.9 (α-helix)	[42]
	Intermediate	168.9 (β-sheet)	20.5 (β-sheet)	[42]
	Fibril	166.9 (β-sheet)	21.5 (β-sheet)	[42]

[*] The structure around each amino acid residues was determined by comparing the experimentally obtained ^{13}C chemical shift values (δ_{iso}) with typical ^{13}C chemical shift values (δ_{iso}) of α-helix and β-sheet, reported as 171.6 and 168.5 for [1-^{13}C]Gly and 14.9 and 19.9 for [3-^{13}C]Ala, respectively [47–49].

Table 1.
Structural transitions during glucagon fibrillation in various conditions as determined by conformation-dependent ^{13}C chemical shifts (ppm)[*].

of glucagon in the fibril state exhibit signals at 167.2 and 21.0 ppm, respectively, and indicate that the vicinities of Gly4 and Ala19 form β-sheet structures.

Conformationally dependent chemical shift values [47–49] clearly indicate that the N-terminus of monomeric glucagon forms an α-helix structure, the center portion forms a random coil, and the C-terminus forms an α-helix structure, as shown in **Table 1** and **Figure 4** (right panels) in acetic acid solution. When the glucagon monomer aggregates to form fibrils, the N-terminal and C-terminal regions change from an α-helix to a β-sheet as seen with other amyloid-forming peptides such as human calcitonin [14] in acetic acid solution.

3. Cytotoxicity of glucagon fibril

The cytotoxicity of the glucagon fibril was assessed by exposing PC12 and NIH-3 T3 cells to 0.1–100 μM peptide aggregate for 72 hrs followed by cell viability determination under the WST-8 assay and released lactate dehydrogenase (LDH) [5]. A significant decrease in cell viability was observed in cultures exposed to 10–100 μM aged glucagon ($P < 0.01$) but not in cultures treated with 100 μM nonaged glucagon. It was determined whether the loss of cell viability was due to cell death by measuring the release of LDH. Treatment with 10 μM aged glucagon induced a significant increase in LDH release compared to control, whereas no significant increase in LDH release was observed in cultures treated with 100 μM nonaged glucagon or 1 μM or lower aged glucagon. Thus, glucagon fibrils were found to be highly toxic to PC12 cells, similar to the case of aged prion protein fragment (PrP)106–126 [50] and β-amyloid (Aβ)1–42 [51] (>10 mM). Aged salmon calcitonin also displayed significant cytotoxicity in PC12 cells, whereas nonaged salmon calcitonin did not induce significant cell death [5].

Next, signaling pathways for the cytotoxicity of peptide fibrils were investigated [5]. Caspase-3 activation is required for the early stages of apoptosis that include DNA fragmentation and morphological changes. To determine whether aged glucagon induces caspase-3 activation in PC12 cells, cells were exposed to 50 μM aged glucagon, and the caspase-3-like activities of the cell lysates were measured by cleavage of the fluorometric caspase-3 substitute Z-DEVD-rhodamine 110. The activity increased prior to the loss of membrane integrity, and 24 hrs after incubation, maximum caspase-3 activity was detected (160% of the control level). In contrast, no significant elevation of casepase-3 activity was observed in cells treated with 50 μM nonaged glucagon. These results indicate that the exposure of PC12 cells to peptide fibrils induces a rapid (within 24 hrs) and significant elevation in casepase-3 activity prior to the loss of cell viability 72 hrs after exposure.

In summary, the misfolding of the therapeutic peptide glucagon generates amyloidogenic fibrils, leading to cytotoxicity mediated by the activation of the apoptotic enzyme caspase-3 in vitro.

4. Kinetic analysis of the glucagon fibrillation process

As shown in **Figure 5**, glucagon monomers (A) first aggregate to form weakly coupled oligomers (A_n) akin to the micelle state. Next, glucagon oligomers (A_n) form fibril intermediates (nuclei) (B_n) through a homogeneous nucleation process with a rate constant k_1. Fibril intermediates (B_n) then react with monomer (A) to form elongated fibrils with a rate constant k_2. This is called the inhomogeneous fibril elongation process. The B form plays a role in the catalysis of A to B, and therefore this is an autocatalytic reaction. Since the nucleation and elongation

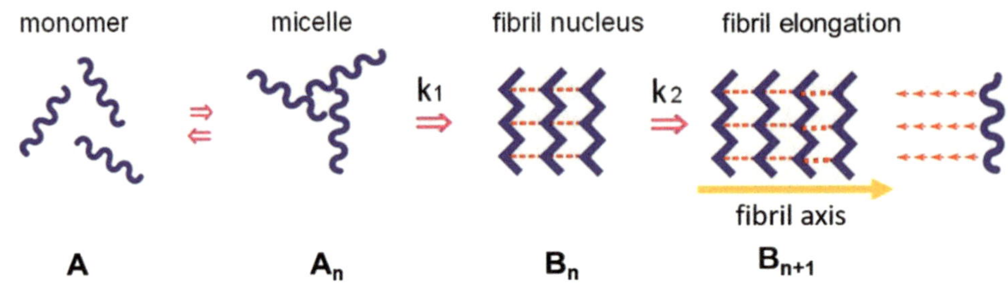

Figure 5.
Schematic of the glucagon fibril formation process in acidic solution. Several monomers (A) aggregate to form weakly coupled micelles (A_n). Micelles (A_n) form a fibril nucleus (B_n) through a homogeneous nucleation process with a rate constant k_1. Fibril nuclei react with monomers (A) to form elongated fibrils (B_{n+1}) with a rate constant k_2. In this reaction, B acts as a catalyst to change the A form to the B form. Overall, this fibril formation reaction is a two-step autocatalytic reaction mechanism.

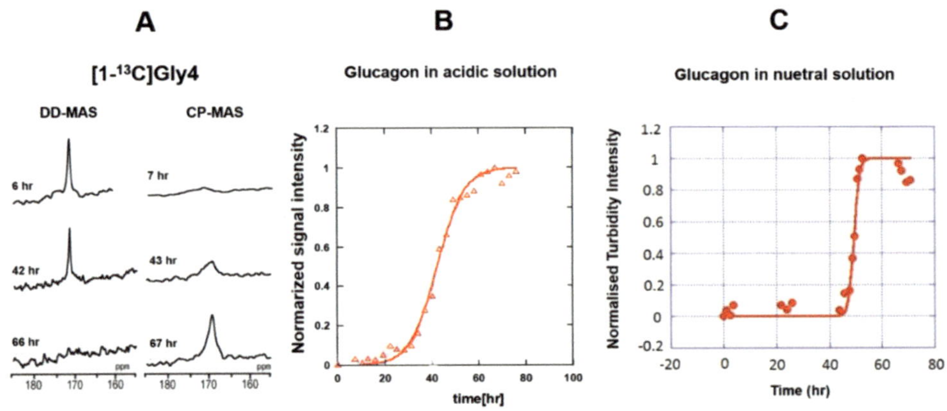

Figure 6.
(A) Time course of changes in the ^{13}C CP-MAS and DD-MAS signals of [1-^{13}C]Gly-glucagon during the fibril formation processes [36]. (B) Plot of normalized CP-MAS signal intensity against elapsed time for glucagon fibril formation in acidic solution at pH 3.3 [36]. (C) Plot of normalized turbidity intensities against elapsed time for glucagon fibril formation in neutral solution (20% acetonitrile solution, pH 7.5) [42].

processes are rate-determining steps, fibril formation is a two-step autocatalytic reaction.

The rate constants of glucagon fibril formation were determined by observing the signal intensities of [1-^{13}C]Gly4 in [1-^{13}C]Gly4 and [3-^{13}C]Ala19-glucagons by ^{13}C CP-MAS NMR spectroscopy with time (**Figure 6A** and **B**). The signal intensities increased after a delay time. The increase in ^{13}C CP-MAS signal intensities corresponds to the increase in fibril components, and thus we obtained the rate constants, k_1 and k_2, for the two-step autocatalytic reaction mechanism, in which k_1 is the rate constant for the fibril nucleation process and k_2 is the rate constant for the fibril elongation process [14].

The first reaction step is homogeneous nuclear formation given by

$$A_{no} \xrightarrow{k_1} B_{no}, \tag{1}$$

where A_{no} is the micelles formed by n_o number of A-form glucagon monomers and B_{no} is the fibrils formed by n_o number of B-form glucagon fibrils. The kinetic equation for Reaction (1) can be given by

$$(df/dt)_1 = k_1(1-f), \tag{2}$$

where f is the fraction of B-glucagon fibrils in the system.

The second heterogeneous fibril elongation reaction can be given by k_2

$$A + B_n \xrightarrow{k_2} B_{n+1}, \tag{3}$$

where B_n and B_{n+1} are elongated fibrils with n and n + 1 number of B-form glucagons. The relevant kinetic equation is given by

$$(df/dt)_2 = k_2 af(1-f), \tag{4}$$

where a is the initial concentration of glucagon. The overall kinetic equation can be given by

$$(df/dt) = (df/dt)_1 + (df/dt)_2 = k_1(1-f) + k_2 a(1-f), \tag{5}$$

Eq. (5) can be integrated to give

$$f = \frac{\rho\{\exp[(1+\rho)kt] - 1\}}{\{1 + \rho\exp[(1+\rho)kt]\}} \tag{6}$$

where f is the fraction of glucagon molecules in the fibril form at time t and ρ represents a dimensionless value describing the ratio of k_1 (the rate constant for the first nucleation process) to k, namely, $\rho = k_1/k$ and $k = ak_2$ (k_2 is the rate constant for the second elongation process of the fibrils, and a is the initial peptide concentration) [14]. The best fits of Eq. (6) are shown in **Figure 6B** (solid lines), and the analyzed rate constants are summarized in **Table 2**. The k_1 and k_2 values were obtained experimentally from the intensity variation of the ^{13}C CP-MAS NMR signals of [1-^{13}C]Gly4 as shown in **Figure 6B** and **Table 2** for glucagon in acidic solution. In comparison, rate constants of fibril formation were obtained for glucagon in neutral solution by plotting the turbidity of the solution against the elapsed time by using an established protocol [52] (**Figure 6C**).

The intensity of the ^{13}C CP-MAS NMR signal of [1-^{13}C]Gly4 was plotted against the elapsed time for glucagon in the presence of bicelles in acidic solution and for glucagon embedded inside lipid bilayers in neutral solution. The obtained rate constants are given in **Table 2**.

Fibril formation condition	k_1 (s^{-1})	k_2 ($s^{-1}M^{-1}$)	Ref.
Acidic solution (0.015 M acetic acid pH 3.3)	2.6×10^{-8}	1.8×10^{-2}	[36]
Neutral solution (20% acetonitrile pH 7.5)	1.2×10^{-24}	4.4×10	[42]
Acidic solution (pH 3.3) in the presence of bicelle (DMPC+DHPC)	2.3×10^{-6}	2.8×10^{-3}	[36]
Inside a lipid bilayer (DMPC) in neutral solution (pH 7.5)	2.8×10^{-7}	5.7×10^{-4}	[42]

Table 2.
Rate constants for glucagon fibril nucleation (k_1) and fibril elongation (k_2) for a two-step autocatalytic reaction mechanism under a variety of conditions.

5. Fibril formation by glucagon in the presence of bicelles in acidic solution

In the presence of bicelles (DMPC-DHPC; 3:1), the N-terminus of glucagon forms an α-helix, the center portion forms a random coil, and the C-terminus forms an α-helix in the monomeric state (**Table 1**). In contrast to glucagon in acetic acid solution, the aggregation of monomers into the fibrils in the presence of bicelles results in the N-terminus maintaining an α-helix structure and the center portion remaining in a random coil structure, whereas the C-terminus changes from an α-helix to a β-sheet structure (**Figure** 7 and **Table 1**). There is therefore significant difference in the structural transition between monomer and fibril in the presence and absence of bicelles, since the N-terminus maintains an α-helix structure in the process of fibril formation in the presence of bicelles. This result suggests that the N-terminal portion of a glucagon fibril significantly interacts with the lipid bilayer surface.

The above findings provide insights into the mechanism of fibril formation in the presence and absence of lipid bilayers, as shown in **Figure** 7. In the absence of lipid bilayers, monomers may aggregate with each other to form oligomeric intermediates (similar to micelles) through a homogeneous reaction (**Figure 7B**; left), likely driven by the amphipathic natures of the N-terminal and C-terminal α-helices. These oligomeric intermediates then change into spherical fibril intermediates (**Figure** 7C; left) as observed by TEM (**Figure 2a** and **b**). Subsequently, these spherical fibril intermediates may form fibril nuclei and interact with monomeric glucagon to allow elongation of the fibril by changing from an α-helix to a β-sheet through a heterogeneous elongation process (**Figure 7D**; left).

In the presence of lipid bilayers, monomers form a structure similar to that in the absence of lipid bilayers. The monomers likely associate quickly with the lipid bilayer and subsequently associate with other monomers to form weakly coupled oligomeric intermediates (**Figure 7B**; right). These oligomeric intermediates may change their structure to form fibril intermediates on the surface of the lipid bilayer and are observed as ellipsoid-shaped fibril intermediates (**Figure 7C**; right and TEM picture) on the surface of the lipid bilayer. The elliptical shape is due to the N-terminal region retaining an α-helix structure even in the fibril intermediates.

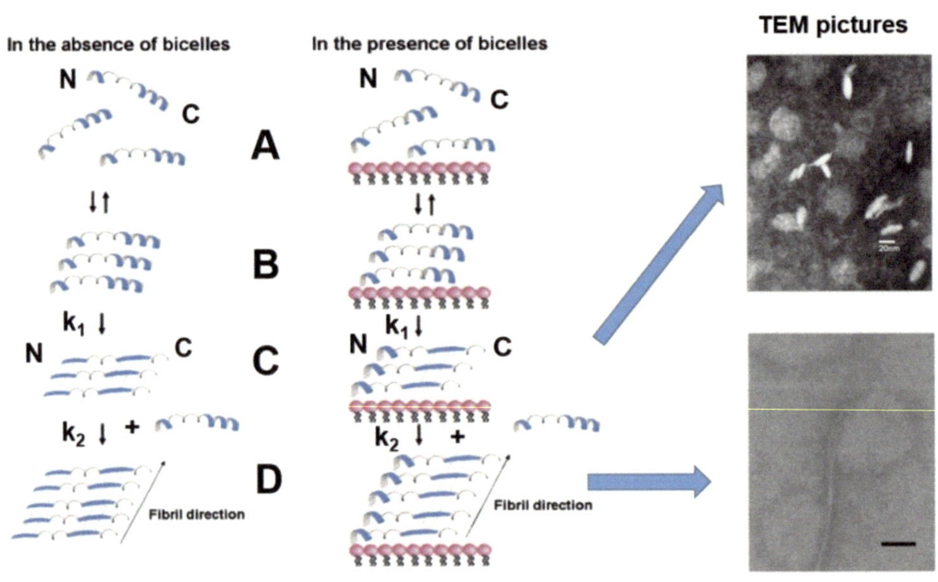

Figure 7.
Schematic diagram of the fibrillation processes of glucagon in acetic acid solution (left) and acidic solution in the presence of bicelles (center). (A) Monomeric form. (B) Weakly coupled oligomer. (C) Fibril intermediate. (D) Elongated fibril. TEM pictures of glucagon fibril intermediates with ellipsoidal shapes and of disk-type bicelles are seen in the top right photo. An elongated fibril is seen attached by its end to a bicelle in the bottom right photo (ref. [36]).

The fibril intermediates grow into longer fibrils on the surface of the lipid bilayer and protrude outside the lipid bilayers, as shown schematically in **Figure 7D** (right) and in the TEM picture (**Figure 7D**; right bottom).

The k_1 rate constant for nuclear formation in the presence of lipid bilayers is faster than in the absence of lipid bilayers (**Table 2**) because glucagon monomers associate with the surface of the lipid bilayer, migrate laterally on the surface of the lipid bilayer to form oligomeric intermediates, and then subsequently change to fibril intermediate through a homogeneous nucleation reaction. This two-dimensional process may be faster than nuclear formation in the three-dimensional solution state.

The k_2 rate constant for fibril elongation in the presence of lipid bilayers is slower than in the absence of lipid bilayers. As discussed previously, the N-terminal part of the glucagon molecule in a fibril in the presence of a lipid bilayer remains in an α-helix which may be stabilized when the helix interacts with the lipid bilayer. However, after the fibril grows and is released from the lipid bilayer, the N-terminal α-helix becomes more unstable than the N-terminal β-sheet formed in a fibril that protrudes from the lipid bilayer. This unstable fibril can grow to the outside of the lipid bilayer because it potentially acts as a template to form structures identical to the fibril nuclei formed on the surface of the lipid bilayer. The instability of the fibril state outside the lipid bilayer results in a decrease in the k_2 value for fibril elongation as compared to the absence of a lipid bilayer.

These results show that glucagon molecules significantly interact with lipid bilayers during the fibril formation processes. To understand the fibril formation process under physiological condition, a variety of lipid bilayer systems including a lipid bilayer in neutral solution were investigated.

6. Fibrillation mechanism of glucagon inside the lipid bilayer in the neutral condition

Fibril formation processes were investigated for glucagon embedded inside a lipid bilayer in neutral solutions (i.e., essentially physiological conditions) [42]. Glucagon-induced morphological changes of lipid bilayers and fibril formation process in a glucagon containing lipid bilayer are shown in **Figure 8**. The monomers may aggregate with each other to form oligomers (**Figure 8B**) likely driven by the amphipathic nature of the N-terminal and C-terminal α-helices. These oligomers then change into ellipsoidal fibril intermediates (nuclei) (**Figure 8C**) through a homogeneous reaction, as observed by TEM (**Figure 8C**, bottom). At this stage, the glucagon intermediates strongly interact with the lipid bilayer to form discoidal lipid bilayer particles. Subsequently, this ellipsoidal fibril intermediate (nucleus) interacts with monomeric glucagon inside the lipid bilayer to allow elongation of the fibril by changing from an α-helix to a β-sheet through a heterogeneous elongation process (**Figure 8D**). After a long time standing, fibril networks are formed, and lipid molecules are compartmentalized (**Figure 8E**), resulting in increased lipid molecule mobility and the induction of a gel-like state throughout the sample, now in an amyloidogenic gel state [53, 54].

The kinetic of fibrillation was thus analyzed using a two-step autocatalytic mechanism as summarized in **Table 2**. The k_1 rate constant for nuclear formation in neutral solution is much slower than that in a DMPC bilayer in neutral conditions (**Table 2**). In a DMPC/glucagon bilayer, glucagon molecules are condensed inside the DMPC bilayer, and thus the nucleation rate of glucagon in a DMPC/glucagon bilayer is much faster than that in neutral solution. The k_1 rate constant for nuclear formation in a lipid bilayer in a neutral solution is slower than in a lipid bilayer in an

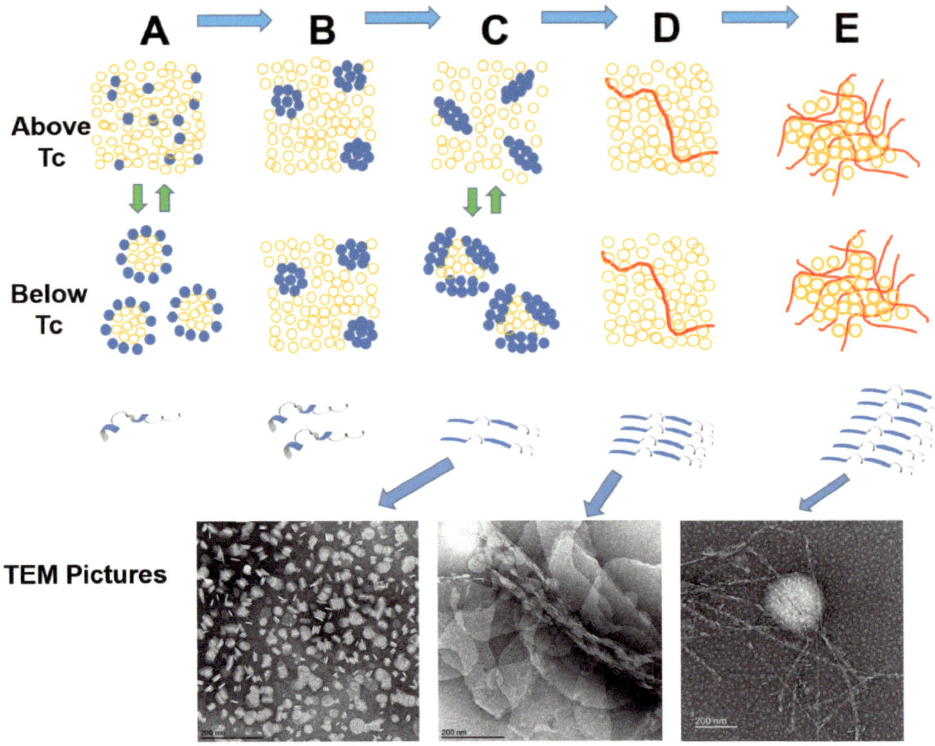

Figure 8.
Schematic diagrams of the morphological states of glucagon-DMPC bilayer systems (DMPC/glucagon; 50/1) at temperatures above and below the phase transition temperature (Tc = 23°C for DMPC). (A) Glucagon-DMPC bilayer state 1 day after sample preparation. (B) Glucagon-DMPC bilayer state 2 days after sample preparation. (C) Glucagon-DMPC bilayer state 4 days after sample preparation with the corresponding TEM picture shown below. (D) Glucagon-DMPC bilayer state 7 days after sample preparation with the corresponding TEM picture shown below. (E) Glucagon-DMPC bilayer system 10 days after sample preparation. The corresponding TEM picture is shown below (ref. [42]).

acidic solution. In an acidic solution, glucagon locates on the surface of lipid bilayer and then migrates laterally on the surface of the lipid bilayer to form oligomers and subsequently changes to fibril nuclei through homogeneous nucleation reaction. In contrast, glucagon is deeply embedded inside a lipid bilayer in neutral solution and thus migrates more slowly inside the lipid bilayer, as reflected in the lower k_1 value.

The k_2 rate constant for the elongation of glucagon fibrils in a DMPC/glucagon bilayer is much slower than that in neutral solution. Glucagon molecules in a DMPC/glucagon bilayer interact strongly with the DMPC bilayer. It therefore takes a long time to disrupt the interaction with the lipid bilayer and form interaction with glucagon fibrils. The k_2 rate constant for fibril elongation in the presence of lipid bilayers under neutral condition is significantly slower than that in lipid bilayers under acidic conditions. Under neutral conditions, glucagon is embedded deep inside the lipid bilayer, and hence it takes longer to release monomeric glucagon from the lipid bilayer. Therefore, the k_2 values for fibril elongation decrease as compared to the case in a lipid bilayer in acidic conditions.

7. Conclusions

It is demonstrated that glucagon forms fibrils in acidic solution and in the presence of lipid bilayer (bicelle) in acidic solution. Glucagon aggregates to form fibril intermediates that glow into elongated fibrils. Glucagon intermediates are formed on the surface of the lipid bilayer in the presence of bicelle. These fibrils are cytotoxic through their activation of apoptotic processes, similar to β-amyloid and salmon calcitonin. Kinetic analyses of glucagon fibril formation are performed using a two-step autocatalytic reaction mechanism comprising fibril nucleation and elongation processes. It is revealed that glucagon forms fibril intermediates and grows into elongated fibrils inside the lipid bilayer under neutral conditions. These properties of glucagon fibril formation indicate that the interaction of the glucagon fibril with lipid bilayers is strongly dependent on the process of fibril formation. A neutral system is thus considered to reflect the fibril formation process in biological cells and provides insight into the mechanism underlying cytotoxicity of glucagon fibrils.

Acknowledgements

This work was supported by Grants-in-Aid for Scientific Research in an Innovative Area (JP16H00756 to AN) and by Grants-in-Aid for Scientific Research (C) (JP15K06963 to AN) from the Ministry of Culture, Sports, Science and Technology of Japan. The author wishes to thank Izuru Kawamura and Yoshiteru Makino for the discussion on this study and Izumi Yamane, Ayano Momose, Hideki Fujita, Eri Yoshimoto, Akie Kikuchi-Kinoshita, and Kazumi Haya for their experimental assistances.

Conflict of interest

The authors declare no conflict of interest.

Author details

Akira Naito
Graduate School of Engineering, Yokohama National University, Yokohama, Japan

*Address all correspondence to: naito@ynu.ac.jp

References

[1] Bromer WW, Sinn LG, Behrens OK. The amino acid sequence of glucagon. V. Location of amide groups, acid degradation studies and summary of sequential evidence. Journal of the American Chemical Society. 1957; **79**:2807-2810. DOI: 10.1021/ja01568a038

[2] Pohl SL, Birnbaumer L, Rodbell M. Glucagon-sensitive adenyl cyclase in plasma membrane of hepatic parenchymal cells. Science. 1969;**164**: 566-567. DOI: 10.1126/science.164.3870

[3] Rodbell M, Birnbaumer L, Pohl SL, Sundby F. The reaction of glucagon with its receptor: Evidence for discrete regions of activity and binding in the glucagon molecule. Proceedings of the National Academy of Sciences of the United States of America. 1971;**68**: 909-913. DOI: 10.1073/pnas.68.5.3870

[4] Beaven GH, Gratzer WB, Davies HG. Formation and structure of gels and fibrils from glucagon. European Journal of Biochemistry. 1969;**11**:37-42. DOI: 10.1111/j.1432.1033.1969.tb00735.x

[5] Onoue S, Ohshima K, Debari K, Koh K, Shioda S, Iwasa S, et al. Mishandling of the therapeutic peptide glucagon generates cytotoxic amyloidogenic fibrils. Pharmaceutical Research. 2004;**21**:1274-1283. DOI: 10.1023/B.PHAM.0000033016.36825.2c

[6] Kamgar-Parsi K, Tolchard J, Habenstein B, Loquet A, Naito A, Ramamoorthy A. Structural biology of calcitonin: From aqueous therapeutic properties to amyloid aggregation. Israel Journal of Chemistry. 2017;**57**:634-650. DOI: 10.1002/ijch.201600096

[7] Burke MJ, Rougvie MA. Cross-β protein structures. I. Insulin fibrils. Biochemistry. 1972;**11**:2435-2439. DOI: 10.1021/bi00763a008

[8] Prusiner SB. Prions. Proceedings of the National Academy of Sciences of the United States of America. 1998;**95**: 13363-13383. DOI: 10.1073/pnas.95.23.13363

[9] Cooper GJS, Willis AC, Clark A, Turner RC, Sim RB, Reid KBM. Purification and characterization of a peptide from amyloid-rich pancreases of type 2 diabetic patients. Proceedings of the National Academy of Sciences of the United States of America. 1987;**84**: 8628-8632. DOI: 10.1073/pnas.95.23.13363

[10] Vines G. Alzheimer's disease – From cause to cure? Trends in Biotechnology. 1993;**11**:49-55. DOI: 10.1016/0167-7799(93)90122-p

[11] Scherzinger E, Lurz R, Turmaine M, Mangiarini L, Hollenbach B, Hasenbank R, et al. Huntington-encoded polyglutamine expansions from amyloid-like protein aggregates in vitro and in vivo. Cell. 1997;**90**: 549-558. DOI: 10.1016/S0092-8674(00)80514-0

[12] Sipe JD. Amyloidosis. Annual Review of Biochemistry. 1992;**61**: 947-975. DOI: 10.1146/annurev.bi.61.070192.004503

[13] Sipe JD, Cohen AS. History of the amyloid fibril. Journal of Structural Biology. 2000;**130**:88-98. DOI: 10.1004/jsbi.2000.4221

[14] Kamihira M, Naito A, Tuzi S, Nosaka AY, Saitô H. Conformational transition and fibrillation mechanism of human calcitonin as studied by high-resolution solid-state ^{13}C NMR. Protein Science. 2000;**9**:867-877. DOI: 10.1110/ps.9.5.867

[15] Itoh-Watanabe H, Kamihira-Ishijima M, Javkhlantugs N, Inoue R,

Itoh Y, Endo H, et al. Role of aromatic residues in amyloid fibril formation of human calcitonin by solid-state ^{13}C NMR and molecular dynamics simulation. Physical Chemistry Chemical Physics. 2013;**15**:8890-8901. DOI: 10.1039/c3cp44544e

[16] Itoh-Watanabe H, Kamihira-Ishijima M, Kawamura I, Kondoh M, Nakakoshi M, Sato M, et al. Characterization of the spherical intermediates and fibril formation of hCT in HEPES solution using solid-state ^{13}C-NMR and transmission electron microscopy. Physical Chemistry Chemical Physics. 2013;**15**:16956-16964. DOI: 10.1039/c3cp52810c

[17] Kamgar-Parsi K, Hong L, Naito A, Brooks CL III, Ramamoorthy A. Growth-incompetent monomers of human calcitonin lead to a noncanonical direct relationship between peptide concentration and aggregation lag time. The Journal of Biological Chemistry. 2017;**292**:14963-14976. DOI: 10.1074/jbcM117.791236

[18] Gorman PM, Chakrabartty A. Alzheimer β-amyloid peptides: Structures of amyloid fibrils and alternate aggregation products. Peptide Science. 2001;**60**:381-394. DOI: 10.1002/1097-0282(2001)60:5<381::AID-BIP/0173>3.0.CO;2-U

[19] Tycko R. Insights into the amyloid folding problem from solid-state NMR. Biochemistry. 2003;**42**:3151-3159. DOI: 10.1021/bi027378p

[20] Tycko R. Application of solid state NMR to the structural characterization of amyloid fibrils: Methods and results. Progress in Nuclear Magnetic Resonance Spectroscopy. 2003;**42**: 53-68. DOI: 10.1016/S0079-6565(03)00003-7

[21] Petkova AT, Yan W-M, Tycko R. Experimental constraints on quaternary structure in Alzheimer's β-amyloid fibrils. Biochemistry. 2006;**45**:498-512. DOI: 10.21/bi051952q

[22] Xiao Y, Ma B, McElheny D, Parthasarathy S, Long F, Hoshi M, et al. Aβ(1-42) fibril structure illuminates self-recognition and replication of amyloid in Alzheimer's disease. Nature Structural & Molecular Biology. 2015; **22**:499-505. DOI: 10.1038/nsmb.2991

[23] Wälti MA, Ravotti F, Arai H, Glabe CG, Wall JS, Böckmann A, et al. Atomic-resolution structure of a disease-relevant Aβ(1-42) amyloid fibril. Proceedings of the National Academy of Sciences of the United States of America. 2016;**113**:E4976-E4984. DOI: 10.1073/pnas1600749113

[24] Colvin MT, Silvers R, Ni QZ, Can TV, Sergeyev I, Rosay M, et al. Atomic resolution structure of monomorphic $A\beta_{42}$ amyloid fibrils. Journal of the American Chemical Society. 2016;**138**:9663-9674. DOI: 10.1021/jacs.6b05129

[25] Sasaki K, Dockerill S, Adamiak DA, Tickle IJ, Blundell T. X-ray analysis of glucagon and its relationship to receptor binding. Nature. 1975;**257**:751-757. DOI: 10.1038/257751a0

[26] Boesch C, Bundi A, Oppliger M, Wüthrich K. ^{1}H nuclear-magnetic-resonance studies of the molecular conformation of monomeric glucagon in aqueous solution. European Journal of Biochemistry. 1978;**91**:209-214. DOI: 10.111/j.1432-1033.1978.tb2095.x

[27] Braun W, Winder G, Lee KH, Wüthrich K. Conformation of glucagon in a lipid-water interphase by ^{1}H nuclear magnetic resonance. Journal of Molecular Biology. 1983;**169**:921-948. DOI: 10.1016/50022-2836(83)80143-0

[28] Onoue S, Iwasa S, Kojima T, Katoh F, Debari K, Koh K, et al.

Structural transition of glucagon in the concentrated solution observed by electrophoretic and spectroscopic techniques. Journal of Chromatography. A. 2006;**1109**:167-173. DOI: 10.1016/j.chroma.2005.11.130

[29] Pedersen JS, Dikov D, Flink JI, Hijuler HA, Christiansen G, Otzen DE. The changing face of glucagon fibrillation: Structural polymorphism and conformational imprinting. Journal of Molecular Biology. 2006;**355**:501-523. DOI: 10.1016/j.jmb.2006.09.100

[30] Pedersen JS, Andersen CB, Otzen DE. Amyloid structure–one but not the same: The many levels of fibrillar polymorphism. FEBS Journal. 2010;**277**: 4591-4601. DOI: 10.1111/j.1742-4658.2010.07888.x

[31] Košmrlj A, Cordsen P, Kyrsting A, Otzen DE, Oddershede LB, Jensen MH. A monomer-trimer model supports intermittent glucagon fibril growth. Scientific Reports. 2015;**5**:9005. DOI: 10.1038/srep09005

[32] Naito A, Kawamura I. Solid-state NMR as a method to reveal structure and membrane-interactions of amyloidogenic protein and peptide. Biochimica et Biophysica Acta. 1768; **2007**:1900-1912. DOI: 10.1016/j.bbamem.2007.03.025

[33] Brender JR, Salamekh S, Ramamoorthy A. Membrane disruption and early events in the aggregation of the diabetes related peptide IAPP from a molecular perspective. Accounts of Chemical Research. 2012;**45**:454-462. DOI: 10.1021/ar200189b

[34] Kotler SA, Walsh P, Brender JR, Ramamoorthy A. Differences between amyloid-β aggregation in solution and on the membrane: Insights into elucidation of the mechanistic details of Alzheimer's disease. Chemical Society Reviews. 2014;**43**:6692-6700. DOI: 10.1039/c3cs60431d

[35] Matsuzaki K. How do membranes initiate Alzheimer's disease? Formation of toxic amyloid fibrils by the amyloid β-protein on ganglioside clusters. Accounts of Chemical Research. 2014; **47**:2397-2404. DOI: 10.1021/ar50012721

[36] Yamane I, Momose A, Fujita H, Yoshimoto E, Kikuchi-Kinoshita A, Kawamura I, et al. Fibrillation mechanism of glucagon in the presence of phospholipid bilayers as revealed by ^{13}C solid-state NMR spectroscopy. Chemistry and Physics of Lipids. 2019; **219**:36-44. DOI: 101016/j.chemphyslip.2019.01.008

[37] Epand RM, Jones AJS, Schreier S. Interaction of glucagon with dimyristoyl glycerophosphocholine. Biochimica et Biophysica Acta. 1977;**491**:296-304. DOI: 10.1016/0005-2795(77)90065-4

[38] Epand RM. Studies on the effect of the lipid phase transition on the interaction of glucagon with dimyristoyl glycerophosphocholine. Biochimica et Biophysica Acta. 1978;**514**:185-197. DOI: 10.1016/0005-2736(78)90290-0

[39] Epand RM, Epand RF, Stewart TP, Hu SW. The condensing effect of glucagon on phospholipid bilayers. Biochimica et Biophysica Acta. 1981; **649**:608-615. DOI: 10.1016/0005-2736(81)90165-6

[40] Naito A, Nagao T, Norisada K, Mizuno T, Tuzi S, Saitô H. Conformation and dynamics of melittin bound to magnetically oriented lipid bilayers by solid-state ^{31}P and ^{13}C NMR spectroscopy. Biophysical Journal. 2000;**78**:2405-2417. DOI: 10.1016/S0006-3495(00)76784-1

[41] Toraya S, Nagao T, Norisada K, Tuzi S, Saitô H, Izumi S. Morphological behavior of lipid bilayers induced by melittin near the phase transition temperature. Biophysical Journal. 2005; **89**:3214-3222. DOI: 10.1529/biophysj.105.059311

[42] Haya K, Makino Y, Kikuchi-Kinoshita A, Kawamura I, Naito A. ^{31}P and ^{13}C Solid-state NMR analysis of morphological changes of phospholipid bilayers containing glucagon during fibril formation of glucagon under neutral condition. Biochim. Biophys. Acta Biomembrane. Forthcoming issue. 2020. DOI: 10.1016/j.bbamem.2020.183290

[43] Andersen CB, Yagi H, Manno M, Martorana V, Ban T, Christiansen G, et al. Branching in amyloid fibril growth. Biophysical Journal. 2000;**96**:1529-1536. DOI: 10.1016/j.bpj.2008.11.024

[44] Andersen CB, Otzen D, Christiansen G, Rischel C. Glucagon amyloid-like fibril morphology is selected via morphology-dependent growth inhibition. Biochemistry. 2007; **46**:7314-7324. DOI: 10.1021.bi6025374

[45] Andersen CB, Hicks MR, Vetri V, Vandahl B, Rahbek-Nielsen H, Thogersen H, et al. Glucagon fibril polymorphism reflects differences in protofilament backbone structure. Journal of Molecular Biology. 2010;**397**: 932-946. DOI: 10.1016/j.jmb.2010.02.012

[46] Jong KLD, Incledon B, Yip CM, DeFelippis MR. Amyloid fibrils of glucagon characterized by high-resolution atomic force microscopy. Biophysical Journal. 2006;**91**:1905-1914. DOI: 10.1529/biophysj.105.077438

[47] Saitô H. Conformation-dependent ^{13}C chemical shifts: A new means of conformation characterization as obtained by high-resolution solid-state ^{13}C NMR. Magnetic Resonance in Chemistry. 1986;**24**:835-852. DOI: 10.1002/mrc.1260241.002

[48] Saitô H, Ando I. High-resolution solid-state NMR studies of synthetic and biological macromolecules. Annual Reports on NMR Spectroscopy. 1989;**21**: 209-290. DOI: 10.1016/50066-4103(08) 60124-6

[49] Saitô H, Ando I, Ramamoorthy A. Chemical shift tensor – The heart of NMR: Insight into biological aspect proteins. Progress in Nuclear Magnetic Resonance Spectroscopy. 2010;**57**: 181-228. DOI: 10.1016/j.pnmrs.2010.04.005

[50] Onoue S, Ohshima K, Endo K, Yajima T, Kashimoto K. PACAP protects neuronal PC12 cells from the cytotoxicity of human prion protein fragment 106-125. FEBS Letters. 2002; **522**:65-72. DOI: 10.1016/50014-5793 (02)02886-7

[51] Onoue S, Endo K, Ohshima K, Yajima T, Kashimoto K. The neuropeptide PACAP attenuates b-amyloid (1-42)-induced toxicity in PC12 cells. Peptides. 2002;**23**:1471-1478. DOI: 10.1016/S0196-9781(02)00085-2

[52] Kamihira-Ishijima M, Nakazawa H, Kira A, Naito A, Nakayama T. Inhibitory mechanism of pancreatic amyloid fibril formation: Formation of the complex between tea catechins and the fragment of residue 22-27. Biochemistry. 2012;**51**:10167-10174. DOI: 10.101021/bi3012274

[53] Azakami H, Mukai A, Kato A. Role of amyloid cross β-structure in the formation of soluble aggregate and gel in heat-induced ovalbumin. Journal of Agricultural and Food Chemistry. 2005; **53**:1254-1257. DOI: 10.1021/jf049325f

[54] Corrigan AM, Donald AM. Particle tracking microrheology of gel-forming amyloid fibril networks. European Physical Journal E: Soft Matter and Biological Physics. 2009;**28**:457-462. DOI: 10.1140/epje/12008-10439-7

Chapter 8

Integrating Nanotherapeutic Platforms to Image Guided Approaches for Management of Cancer

Asad Ali, Zeeshan Ahmad, Usama Ahmad, Mohd Muazzam Khan, Md. Faheem Haider and Juber Akhtar

Abstract

Cancer is a leading cause of mortality worldwide, accounting for 8.8 million deaths in 2015. The landscape of cancer therapeutics is rapidly advancing with development of new and sophisticated approaches to diagnostic testing. Treatment plan for early diagnosed patients include radiation therapy, tumor ablation, surgery, immunotherapy and chemotherapy. However the treatment can only be initiated when the cancer has been diagnosed thoroughly. Theranostics is a term that combines diagnostics with therapeutics. It embraces multiple techniques to arrive at comprehensive diagnosis, molecular images and an individualized treatment regimen. Recently, there is an effort to tangle the emerging approach with nanotechnologies, in an attempt to develop theranostic nanoplatforms and methodologies. Theranostic approach to management of cancer offers numerous advantages. They are designed to monitor cancer treatment in real time. A wide variety of theranostic nanoplatforms that are based on diverse nanostructures like magnetic nanoparticles, carbon nanotubes, gold nanomaterials, polymeric nanoparticles and silica nanoparticles showed great potential as cancer theranostics. Nano therapeutic platforms have been successful in integrating image guidance with targeted approach to treat cancer.

Keywords: nanomedicine, theranostics, targeted delivery, cancer, functionalized nanomedicine

1. Introduction

Cancer has a major impact on society across the world. Estimated number of new cases of cancer, current cases of cancer, deaths, survival rate, mortality and in depth information, symptoms of cancer, its early detection, prevention and treatment all are provided by American Cancer Society. Nearly 13% of cancer diagnosed in 2017 was in the young at age of 20. The new review statistics shows 28 types of rare cancer which talks about mortality rate, survival, diagnosis and also provides an idea about symptoms and risk factors related to different types of cancer [1].

Therapeutic approaches such as development of nanoemulsions, liposomes, microspheres and nanoparticles have facilitated in fighting cancer. Among these, the simplest platforms are the nanoemulsion having size range of 100 to 500 nm which are kinetically stabilized having high content of oil and low amount of surfactant [2]. Solubility of poorly soluble drugs [3, 4] and its bioavailability can be increased by converting the drug into forms like capsule and gels [5] or can be used in their original form. The method used for the fabrication of nanoemulsion are high energy methods (microfluidization and sonication) and low energy emulsification method [6–8].

Theranostics is a term originally coined to define an approach that combine's diagnostics with therapeutics [9]. It embraces multiple techniques to arrive at comprehensive diagnosis, molecular images and an individualized treatment regimen [10, 11]. Recently, there is an effort to tangle the emerging approach with nanotechnologies, in an attempt to develop theranostic nanoplatforms and methodologies [12]. Given that cancer is a highly heterogeneous and adaptable disease, diverse types of treatment options need to be chosen depending on patient's characteristics and disease progression.

2. Theranostics

Drugs or methods that are used for accompanying diagnosis and cure [13] are referred to as Theranostics. One of the achievements of nanotechnology is the fabrication of theranostic nanomedicine for the preparation of these types of drugs. The term defines "a nanotherapeutic system which can deliver targeted therapy and diagnose". This aspect provides help when fabricating nano based image contrasting agent and also in image guided therapeutics [14].

Rapid drug development, advanced disease management, reduced associated risk and cost are assumed to be the result of mutual techniques. Such type of investigation which involves quick diagnosis and treatment are very helpful in disease which are a major cause of morbidity and/or mortality and cancer is one of the disease and coincidently the initial research in theranostic is dedicated to oncology. Sound knowledge, core understanding of detection and therapy mechanism are required for the formation of theranostic agents. In order to fabricate theranostic agents one should have understanding of diagnostic strategies, molecular mechanism adverse effect and toxicity of material and techniques for nanoparticles preparation for therapy and diagnostic purpose.

Research in theranostics has rapidly improved in the past decade resulting into preparation of different contrast media and active ingredient with different method of preparation. Preparation of dual purpose nanoparticle system is the main aim of theranostics. Therefore it is important to put attention on all factors that influences the process, right from the preparation of nanoemulsion/nanoparticle till the removal of metabolites of the active molecules and other materials used. The factors can be the compatibility between chemicals, the condition in which the formulation is prepared, modification in formulations because of selected route of administration, the toxicity, metabolites of active ingredient, its biocompatibility and biodegradability and evaluation of pharmacodynamic and pharmacokinetic parameter and eventually the disadvantage and benefits of the process.

The basis of diagnosis in theranostics depends upon using different contrast agent during imaging. MRI is the most studied and used technique among all different imaging mechanism and a lot has been spent on research related to magnetic particles used as contrasting agent. Metals like gold, silver, iron oxide have been studied with the object of finding suitable particle for imaging with least toxicological effect. Diseased tissue and healthy tissue are differentiated in MRI by the use of these particles.

Contrast agent	Drug used	Applications	Size	Zeta potential	References
Manganese oxide	siRNA	MRI plus RNA delivery	—	—	[15]
Gold	DOX Diagnosis	tumor targeting and PTT	45.97 nm and 6.3 nm	−3.54 mV	[16–18]
Iron oxide	siRNA, DOX, docetaxel	Targeting, MRI and therapy	30 nm	−5 mV	[19–21]
Silica	Pyropheophorbide (HPPH), DOX	Drug carrier, X-ray/CT imaging, Photodynamic therapy	30 nm and 126 nm	−39 mV	[22, 23]
CNTs	DNA plasmid, DOX, PTX	Diagnosis, DNA and drug delivery	20 nm and 120.6 nm	—	[24, 25]
QDs	DOX, MTX	Imaging, therapy and sensing	—	—	[26]

Abbreviations: siRNA: short interfering ribonucleic acid, CNTs: carbon nanotubes, QDs: quantum dots, DOX: Doxorubicin, HPPH: 2-[1-hexyloxyethyl]-2-devinyl pyropheophorbide-alpha, MTX: Methotrexate, PTX: Paclitaxel, MRI: Magnetic resonance imaging, CT: Computed topography.

Table 1.
Different theranostic agents used for biomedical applications.

As stated one of the brutal disease is cancer and hence theranostic research has put an eye on this area. Day by day the research is going on in positive direction and much useful research has already been carried out. In order to understand the concept of diagnosis of cancer and therapy related to it the use of nanoparticle agents is in progression [27, 28]. One such example of theranostic agent is manganese oxide nanoparticle carrying drugs and contrast agents [29] and silica nanoparticle with magnetic and fluorescent tags [30]. In the past few years, combination of metal nanoparticle or shells [31–33] with magnetic components has yielded different theranostic agents for biomedical applications which are widely used. Some examples of theranostic agents are given in **Table 1**.

3. Nano theranostics

Theranostic nanosystems comprise of platforms/nanocarriers that are used as imaging as well as therapeutic agents via a single entity. Nanotheranostic devices can be made by many types of inorganic and organic nanomaterials. Preclinical implementations make use of nanotheranostic system because they might provide a way or method of understanding many crucial aspects of drug delivery and how these systems can assist in knowing the power of personalized medicines.

4. Therapeutic agents

At present radiotherapy, surgery and chemotherapy are possible treatments for cancer patients. The purpose of the theranostic is to use these therapeutic strategies and reduce the risk associated with chemotherapy and radiotherapy and in addition to it avoid complications related to surgery and trauma. In addition, with the help of nanotechnology, theranostics may support the diversification of therapeutic approaches like PTT, PDT and immunotherapy. Here we report some of these therapeutic strategies often used in theranostics, like radiotherapy, chemotherapy, PDT, PTT and immunotherapy.

5. Chemotherapy for management of cancer

Anticancer drugs have proven beneficial in improving survival rate of cancer patients [34]. There are huge numbers of clinical anti-cancer drugs which are broadly applied to theranostics. On the basis of structure and resource of chemotherapy drugs, cancer therapeutic agents can be classified into six types: alkylating agent, antitumor antibiotic, phytogenic anticarcinogen, antimetabolites, hormone and miscellaneous anti-cancer drugs. Thermo DOX for liver cancer, Doxil for ovarian cancer therapy and Myocet for metastatic breast cancer are few cancer nanomedicines that have been approved by the FDA. Theranostic systems also make use of prodrugs like platinum (IV) prodrug to reduce the toxicity of drug and by increasing the active hits to the cells of tumors site. Due to their broad availability these prodrugs are very popular option. The UV light is transformed from NIR light by UCNP which activates the prodrugs to highly toxic platinum (II) complexes that enters the cell by endocytosis after grafted onto up converting nanoparticles (UCNP) [35]. In order to attain best therapeutic efficacy of drug delivery systems a high payload is essential. In theranostics, in order to maintain the original size and solubility in aqueous media a carrier with large pore volume and surface area are given preferences so that more therapeutic agent can be carried [36]. For example, Sorafenib with a loading ration of 28.2% can be loaded on porous silica nanoparticles and may release the therapeutic agent in sustained fashion [37]. GO, Ws2 and MoS2 are some of the popular 2-D nanomaterials that have a very high drug payload as they can bear chemotherapeutics on both sides of sheet. Some of the example of high drug payload include 118% for 7-ethyl-10-hydroxycamptothecin (SN38) and approx 239% for DOX were observed on MoS2 [38], DOX (approximately 400%) on GO [39] was also significant. Cancer cells show multidrug resistance (MDR) often when they are treated by single drug which can be overcome by employing efficient strategies of theranostics. By combining P-glycoprotein (P-gp) reversing agent with anticancer drug the hurdle of MDR can be resolved [40]. The function of P-gp reversing agent is to avoid the pumping of chemotherapeutic drugs out of cancer cells due to over expression of P-gp. One way to overcome MDR is by covering the positive change that is present on anticancer drugs. DOX alone cannot produce significant cancer effect but when it is adsorbed on the surface of polymeric nanoparticle more chance are there that cancer cell may readily uptake it and accumulate within cancer cell and produce more cytotoxicity to cancer cell. Nanocarriers loaded with combination of anticancer drugs provide synergistic effect thereby improving overall management of cancer [41, 42].

6. Photothermal therapy for management of cancer

Microwave, light irradiation or magnetic field can potentiate the effect of thermal therapy which in turn employs hyperthermia to kill cancer cells. Among all the above mentioned therapies photothermal therapy has the maximum capacity to destroy cancer cell while causing least damage to nearby healthy cells. Localized hyperthermia under light irradiation at tumor site is generated by using NIR absorbing agent in photothermal therapy [43]. In MR region an ideal PTT agent should show strong absorbance and must exhibit less fluorescence quantum yield thereby promoting efficient conversion of absorbed light energy into heat via non-radiative transition rather than fluorescence emission.

Inorganic nanoparticles and organic dyes are extensively employed as PTT agents. Examples of organic dyes include Prussian blue, IR780, ICG, IR820, Cypate, IR825. These organic dyes have an added advantage of ease of loading on nanoplatforms and ideal NIR absorbance [44]. In order to improve the photostability and targeting ability of organic dyes they are being encapsulated into nanocarriers [45]. Carbocyanine dyes namely cypate and ICG were loaded into the polymeric micelle with loading rate of 50% and 20% for cypate and ICG respectively. Upon comparing loaded theranostic polymeric micelle with carbocyanine dye alone showed marked cellular uptake and longer retention time at the site of tumor. Remarkable PTT results were observed along with increased photothermal effect and photostability of organic dyes when nanomaterials like graphene derivatives absorbing strongly in the NIR regions were employed [46]. In NIR and PTT imaging techniques both cypate and ICG can be used as theranostic agents.

Photothermal conversion efficiency will decrease in presence of high fluorescence quantum yield and fluorescence imaging is disturbed in case of low quantum yield hence there is not much surety in theranostic application of organic dyes. Apart from the organic dyes, a wide range of inorganic nanoparticles have been fabricated for theranostic applications. Inorganic nanoparticles exhibit strong photothermal conversion efficiency and NIR absorption for PTT. It encompasses customized gold nanostructure like nanoshell, nanocages, nanorods and nanotubes. On comparing the gold nanorods alone against gold nanorods coated with Pt nanodots, the latter showed significant better photothermal effect than the former [47]. And the better results were due to the presence of Pt shell in the endosomes which not only prevented the original sharp LSPR band of gold nanorods from shifting and dampening but also prevented the aggregation of gold nanorods. Carbon nanotubes [48], carbon dots [49], GO are some of the other nanomaterials that can used for PTT. GO for in-vivo PTT was used for the first time by Liu group. Further they reduced the GO to rGO which had 7 times more NIR absorption than GO hence increasing the PTT effect [50]. PTT for now might only be used for treating skin cancer and not for internal cancer because of limiting light penetration depth but its noteworthy therapeutics capacities with minimum possible side effect cannot be ignored. Further study is required to get deeper insight about how phototoxicity is caused by PTT.

Apart from PTT, hyperthermia induced magnetically is also one of the non-invasive procedures to treat cancer [51]. Dielectric constant and microwave frequency between malignant tissue and normal tissue in breast can be employed for the detection and treatment of breast cancer. Dielectric contrast is used for scattering of an illuminating microwave signal and the incident microwave produces hyperthermia thereby treating malignant tissues [52].

7. Photodynamic therapy for management of cancer

Photosensitizers (PSs) used in PDT plays a vital role in the treatment of cancer and possess enormous potential. Cytotoxic reactive oxygen species or free radicals are generated when the molecular oxygen surrounding the diseased cell reacts with the absorbed light that is being transferred by PSs under laser irradiation which finally causes cell apoptosis and damage to cancerous cells [53]. No side effects are observed from photosensitizes and generate ROS only when laser light is irradiated upon them.

PDT requires low light density to cause damage to cancer cell unlike the PTT which requires high density laser light to generate hyperthermia that can cause damage to cancer cells [54]. PDT encompasses noteworthy advantages like very less invasiveness, on repeating the therapy is show no cumulative toxicity, very less damage to immune and hemopoietic system thereby improving the overall health and contributing to quality life for the patient. An ideal PS must have following properties like triplet state formation of high quantum yield and a good amount of triplet lifetime so that interaction with ground state oxygen is possible thereby generating sufficient ROS. However many PSs does not have good tumor selectivity, good amount of photosensitivity and absorption maxima above 700 nm [55]. A distinctive NIR absorption at 700 nm was observed by the help of extra axial mob linkers in monosubstituted phthalocyanine [56] that produced 20 nm red shift of characteristic Q band. PEG functionalized iron oxide nanocluster surface when loaded with Ce6 the absorption peak of chlorine e6 (Ce6) showed red shift from 650 nm to 704 nm [57]. The energy transferred from UCNPs to PSs are able to excite the combination of PSs and UCNP's, therefore inhibiting the growth of tumor by generation of cytotoxic singlet oxygen [58].

8. Radiation therapy for management of cancer

Radiation therapy has become an integral part to treat many sarcomas. The mechanism of action of radiation therapy is that the radiation damages strings of DNA in the nucleus of cells which stops the cell multiplication. Apart from aforementioned functions of radiation therapy, it also produces reactive oxygen therapy (ROS) which indirectly damages the tumor cell and also damages the DNA of mitochondria and other organelle of cell. In case of surgical resection, the survival could be prolonged by employing radiation therapy. However due to frequent and repeated high dose of X-ray irradiation that causes systemic side effects and resistance to radiation had been noticed in cancerous cells.

Metal nanoparticles in strong association with strong capacities of photoelectric absorbance are used as radiation dose enhancing agents. For example research shows that radio sensitization is being mediated by Gold NP due to greater energy deposition and absorption in surrounding tissue from photoelectrons. Radiotherapy with prolonged circulation time in blood has been demonstrated by Auger electrons and characteristic X-rays [59] and polyethylene glycosylation modified gold nanoparticle (N GNPs). Radiotherapy can relieve the symptoms and prolong the lives of terminal cancer patients. However radiotherapy is not an easy task and may cause loss of organ functions also as it may also induce many complications. Moreover, it cannot completely remove cancer cells. In coming future we may see highly accurate and precise exposure of tumor site to high radiation by the application of radiation wave knife for much better clinical results.

9. Immunotherapy for management of cancer

After radiotherapy, surgery or chemotherapy it has been observed that a small number of cancer cells may still remain alive and in addition to it the overall treatment quality is also decreased due to drug resistance. Immunotherapy has great potential to treat cancer as it acts on the immune system rather than on the tumor itself. Immunotherapy is considered as a unique and promising strategy for cancer therapy [60] and the main advantages include its specific promotion on immune cells only aiming on target cells or target tissues. So far, the related investigations have been gradually transformed from laboratory research to clinical practice. For clinical treatment the use of immunotherapeutic drugs such as immune checkpoint inhibitors and T cells have been approved by FDA and have great potential for cancer treatment. Improved immunotherapeutic nanomaterials loaded with antigens, immune adjuvants and nucleic acids have been demonstrated to be helpful. The nanoplatforms may affect and alter immune cell actions and response non-specifically. They may easily damage the cancer cells and achieve tumor targeting with pathogens factors. For e.g. repetitive and homogenous antigens conjugated with gold nanoparticles are able to trigger immune response in an in-vitro setting even without the use of adjuvant. Recently a combination of IR phthalocyanine dye IR700 with monoclonal antibodies had been fabricated and this novel technique is known as Photoimmunotherapy [61]. Least side effect and significantly fast cell necrosis rate is observed when antibodies bind to target tumor cells during the PIT and is activated by NIR light irradiation. Hence for monitoring and treating cancer in a highly selective manner PIT is a good theranostic approach.

10. Multimodal therapy for management of cancer

Conventional cancer therapies often do not succeed to eradicate tumor completely. In order to recover anticancer efficacy, the arrangement of two or more therapeutic modalities such as chemo photodynamic, photothermal photodynamic, chemo photo thermal synergistic formulations have been explored. Thermomotherapeutic characteristics in association with theranostic methods result in development of anticancer drug that possess synergistic therapeutic effect [62]. Chemotherapy could be improved by the use of photothermal effect which aids the intracellular translocation of anti-cancer drugs [63]. Risk of overtreatment could be minimized along with the reduction in dose of therapeutic agent with less laser exposure time. All these can be attained by combination of PDT/PTT. Synergistic effect of PTT/PDT have been seen when GO was loaded with methylene blue [64]. In this system, lesser dose of nano GO was applied, as compared to the particular PTT treatment of nano GO. In addition, the PTT and PDT combinational treatment could be spoil both superficial and deep regions of the tumor, and thus overcome the drawbacks of single treatments [65]. To further progress cancer therapy efficacy, numerous types of theranostic platforms were developed to combine chemotherapy, PTT and PDT simultaneously [66]. Treating cancer with combinational therapy has become an essential trend in cancer therapeutics. Compared to single modality therapy, the combined therapy can reduce the dosage of the drugs and thus decrease the side effects in treatment. More prominently, the combined therapy has the potential to decrease multidrug resistance of tumor cells, thus improving the therapeutic efficacy. The combined therapy may bring a novel opportunity to the next invention of cancer treatment [67].

11. Imaging-guided therapy for management of cancer

The theranostic nanoparticles have an ever increasing consideration for image guided therapy in current years because these nanoparticles can follow the pharmacokinetic process, guide the treatment and monitor therapeutic process and outcome. They could be employed to imagine and quantify the performance of drug delivery systems for numerous special purposes such as biodistribution and pharmacokinetics of nanocarriers, metabolic response and drug release process of the nanocarriers. Koukourakis group and Harrington group engaged Technetium

Imaging method	Imaging agent	Therapeutic agent	Function
Optical Imaging	Cy5.5	Paclitaxel	Real time tracking of NP location
	FITC-coumarin pair	Doxorubicin	Drug release monitoring
	Dicyanomethylene-4H-pyran	Camptothecin	Drug release monitoring
	Cy7, 111In	Cyclophosphamide, etoposide	Real time imaging of apoptosis
	Cy5.5-BHQ pair	Doxorubicin	Real time imaging of apoptosis
	Ce6	Ce6	Real time tracking of NP location & PDT
	Ce6-BHQ pair	Ce6	Drug release monitoring & PDT
	UCNP (β-NaYF4:Yb3+,Er3+)	Cisplatin prodrug	Imaging of NP location
	UCNP (NaYF4:Er)	TPGSd	Dual imaging (optical, CT) & reducing multidrug resistance
	UCNP (NaYF4:Yb/Er)	Ce6, doxorubicin	Imaging of particle location & chemotherapy/PDT
MR imaging	Gd	Doxorubicin	Real time monitoring of drug delivery
	SPION	SPION	Detection & hyperthermia treatment of tumor
	SPION	Doxorubicin	Tumor detection & chemotherapy
	SPION/FITC	siRNA	MR imaging & gene therapy
CT imaging	GNP	Doxorubicin	CT imaging of cancer & chemotherapy
	GNR	GNR	Dual imaging (X-ray/CT) & PTT/radio sensitization
PET Imaging	64Cu	Doxorubicin	Quantitative biodistribution analysis & Chemotherapy
	64Cu	siRNA	Quantitative determination of biodistribution & efficacy of siRNA NPs
US imaging	Perfluoropentane	Docetaxel	Triggered drug release & chemotherapy
	CaCO3	Doxorubicin	Tumor imaging & triggered drug release
	Perfluorooctyl bromide	Camptothecin	Chemotherapy & ablation therapy
	Perfluorohexane	CPT11m	Tumor imaging & chemotherapy/ablation Therapy

Table 2.
Theranostic technologies for cancer treatment [68].

and Indium labeled PEGylated liposomes respectively to monitor drug targeting to the sarcomas and breast cancer sites [69]. In the clinical practice, surgical resection is a regular and inevitable procedure for cancer therapy. Theranostics gives a possibility in intraoperative imaging to guide the operation process. During the surgery, physicians could congregate the diagnostic information for precise imaging as well as visualized therapy. In theranostic platform, DOTA-Gd act as a MRI contrast agent for preoperative finding and surgical planning; the Raman molecules visualized the excellent margin of tumor, allowing precise resection for the duration of operation process. The multimodal NP could recognize tumor edge for precise resection of tumor. This approach could be planned for simple intraoperative navigation and real-time imaging [70]. Theranostic technologies commonly utilized for cancer treatment are given in **Table 2**.

12. Conclusion

Theranostic approach to management of cancer offers numerous advantages. They are designed to monitor cancer treatment in real time. A wide variety of theranostic nanoplatforms that are based on diverse nanostructures like magnetic nanoparticles, carbon nanotubes, gold nanomaterials, polymeric nanoparticles, or silica nanoparticles showed great potential as cancer theranostics. Nano therapeutic platforms have been successful in integrating image guidance with targeted approach to treat cancer.

Conflict of interest

Authors declare no conflict of interest related to this manuscript.

Abbreviations

PTT	Photothermal therapy
PDT	Photodynamic therapy
DOX	Doxorubicin
NIR	Near infrared
MRI	Magnetic resonance imaging
PET	Positron emission tomography
CT	Computed topography
UNCPs	Up converting nanoparticles
GO	Grapheme oxide
MDR	Multidrug resistance
MoS_2	Molybdenum disulfide
ICG	Indocyanine green
WS_2	Tungsten disulfide
Ce6	Chlorine e6

Author details

Asad Ali[1], Zeeshan Ahmad[2], Usama Ahmad[1]*, Mohd Muazzam Khan[1], Md. Faheem Haider[1] and Juber Akhtar[1]

1 Faculty of Pharmacy Integral University, Lucknow, India

2 Makams Industries Private Limited, Bhiwadi, Alwar, Rajasthan, India

*Address all correspondence to: usamaahmad.10@outlook.com

References

[1] https://www.cancer.org/research/cancer-facts-statistics/all-cancer-facts-figures/cancer-facts-figures-2017.html (last accessed on 01/08/2020)

[2] McClements DJ. Nanoemulsions versus microemulsions: Terminology, differences, and similarities. Soft Matter. 2012;**8**(6):1719-1729

[3] Ahmad, U., Akhtar, J., Singh, S.P., Badruddeen, Ahmad, F.J., Siddiqui, S. and Wahajuddin, 2017. Silymarin nanoemulsion against human hepatocellular carcinoma: development and optimization. Artificial cells, nanomedicine, and biotechnology, 46(2), pp.231-241.

[4] Shakeel F, Shafiq S, Haq N, Alanazi FK, Alsarra IA. Nanoemulsions as potential vehicles for transdermal and dermal delivery of hydrophobic compounds: An overview. Expert Opinion on Drug Delivery. 2012;**9**(8):953-974

[5] Sarker DK. Engineering of nanoemulsions for drug delivery. Current Drug Delivery. 2005;**2**(4):297-310

[6] Ali A, Ansari VA, Ahmad U, Akhtar J, Jahan A. Nanoemulsion: An advanced vehicle for efficient drug delivery. Drug research. 2017;**67**(11):617-631

[7] Constantinides PP, Chaubal MV, Shorr R. Advances in lipid nanodispersions for parenteral drug delivery and targeting. Advanced Drug Delivery Reviews. 2008;**60**(6):757-767

[8] Maali A, Mosavian MH. Preparation and application of nanoemulsions in the last decade (2000-2010). Journal of Dispersion Science and Technology. 2013 Jan 1;**34**(1):92-105

[9] Chen XS. Introducing theranostics journal-from the editor-in-chief. Theranostics. 2011;**1**:1

[10] Lukianova-Hleb EY, Oginsky AO, Samaniego AP, Shenefelt DL, Wagner DS, Hafner JH, et al. Tunableplasmonicnanoprobes for theranostics of prostate cancer. Theranostics. 2011;**1**:3

[11] Zhu L, Xie J, Swierczewska M, Zhang F, Quan Q, Ma Y, et al. Real-time video imaging of protease expression in vivo. Theranostics. 2011;**1**:18

[12] Fang C, Zhang M. Nanoparticle-based theragnostics: Integrating diagnostic and therapeutic potentials in nanomedicine. Journal of Controlled Release: Official Journal of the Controlled Release Society. 2010;**146**(1):2

[13] Ahmed N, Fessi H, Elaissari A. Theranostic applications of nanoparticles in cancer. Drug Discovery Today. 2012;**17**(17-18):928-934

[14] Sumer, B. and Gao, J., 2008. Theranosticnanomedicine for Cancer.

[15] Bae KH, Lee K, Kim C, Park TG. Surface functionalized hollow manganese oxide nanoparticles for cancer targeted siRNA delivery and magnetic resonance imaging. Biomaterials. 2011;**32**(1):176-184

[16] Huang P, Bao L, Zhang C, Lin J, Luo T, Yang D, et al. Folic acid-conjugated silica-modified gold nanorods for X-ray/CT imaging-guided dual-mode radiation and photo-thermal therapy. Biomaterials. 2011;**32**(36):9796-9809

[17] Chen W, Bardhan R, Bartels M, Perez-Torres C, Pautler RG, Halas NJ, et al. A molecularly targeted theranostic probe for ovarian cancer. Molecular Cancer Therapeutics. 2010;**9**(4):1028-1038

[18] Prabaharan M, Grailer JJ, Pilla S, Steeber DA, Gong S. Gold nanoparticles

with a monolayer of doxorubicin-conjugated amphiphilic block copolymer for tumor-targeted drug delivery. Biomaterials. 2009;**30**(30):6065-6075

[19] Lee JH, Lee K, Moon SH, Lee Y, Park TG, Cheon J. All-in-one target-cell-specific magnetic nanoparticles for simultaneous molecular imaging and siRNA delivery. AngewandteChemie. 2009;**121**(23):4238-4243

[20] Yang K, Zhang S, Zhang G, Sun X, Lee ST, Liu Z. Graphene in mice: Ultrahigh in vivo tumor uptake and efficient photothermal therapy. Nano Letters. 2010;**10**(9):3318-3323

[21] Ling Y, Wei K, Luo Y, Gao X, Zhong S. Dual docetaxel/superparamagnetic iron oxide loaded nanoparticles for both targeting magnetic resonance imaging and cancer therapy. Biomaterials. 2011;**32**(29):7139-7150

[22] RoyI, OhulchanskyyTY, PudavarHE, Bergey EJ, Oseroff AR, Morgan J, et al. Ceramic-based nanoparticles entrapping water-insoluble photosensitizing anticancer drugs: A novel drug– carrier system for photodynamic therapy. Journal of the American Chemical Society. 2003;**125**(26):7860-7865

[23] Park JH, Gu L, Von Maltzahn G, Ruoslahti E, Bhatia SN, Sailor MJ. Biodegradable luminescent porous silicon nanoparticles for in vivo applications. Nature Materials. 2009;**8**(4):331

[24] Pantarotto D, Singh R, McCarthy D, Erhardt M, Briand JP, Prato M, et al. Functionalized carbon nanotubes for plasmid DNA gene delivery. AngewandteChemie. 2004;**116**(39):5354-5358

[25] Liu Z, Chen K, Davis C, Sherlock S, Cao Q, Chen X, et al. Drug delivery with carbon nanotubes for in vivo cancer treatment. Cancer Research. 2008;**68**(16):6652-6660

[26] Savla R, Taratula O, Garbuzenko O, Minko T. Tumor targeted quantum dot-mucin 1 aptamer-doxorubicin conjugate for imaging and treatment of cancer. Journal of Controlled Release. 2011;**153**(1):16-22

[27] Li Z, Chen H, Bao H, Gao M. One-pot reaction to synthesize water-soluble magnetite nanocrystals. Chemistry of Materials. 2004;**16**(8):1391-1393

[28] Souza KC, Salazar-Alvarez G, Ardisson JD, Macedo WAA, Sousa EMB. Mesoporoussilica–magnetitenanocomposite synthesized by using a neutral surfactant. Nanotechnology. 2008;**19**(18):185603

[29] Liong M, Lu J, Kovochich M, Xia T, Ruehm SG, Nel AE, et al. Multifunctional inorganic nanoparticles for imaging, targeting, and drug delivery. ACS Nano;**2**(5):2008, 889-2896

[30] Insin N, Tracy JB, Lee H, Zimmer JP, Westervelt RM, Bawendi MG. Incorporation of iron oxide nanoparticles and quantum dots into silica microspheres. ACS Nano. 2008;**2**(2):197-202

[31] Kang L-J et al. Stabilization of superparamagnetic iron oxide core–gold shell nanoparticles in high ionic strength media. Langmuir. 2009;**25**:13384

[32] Zhao N, Gao M. Magnetic janus particles prepared by a flame synthetic approach: Synthesis, characterizations and properties. Advanced Materials. 2009;**21**(2):184-187

[33] Kamei K, Mukai Y, Kojima H, Yoshikawa T, Yoshikawa M, Kiyohara G, et al. Direct cell entry of gold/iron-oxide magnetic nanoparticles in adenovirus mediated gene delivery. Biomaterials. 2009;**30**(9):1809-1814

[34] Wang L, Qiao H, Han J, Chen Y, Wang D, Li D. The mutual beneficial effect between medical imaging and nanomedicine. Journal of Nanomaterials. 2013;**2013**:5

[35] Dai Y, Xiao H, Liu J, Yuan Q, Ma PA, Yang D, et al. In vivo multimodality imaging and cancer therapy by near-infrared light-triggered trans-platinum pro-drug-conjugated upconverison nanoparticles. Journal of the American Chemical Society. 2013;**135**(50):18920-18929

[36] Chen F, Hong H, Zhang Y, Valdovinos HF, Shi S, Kwon GS, et al. In vivo tumor targeting and image-guided drug delivery with antibody-conjugated, radiolabeled mesoporous silica nanoparticles. ACS Nano. 2013;**7**(10):9027-9039

[37] Wang CF, Sarparanta MP, Mäkilä EM, Hyvönen ML, Laakkonen PM, Salonen JJ, et al. Multifunctional porous silicon nanoparticles for cancer theranostics. Biomaterials. 2015;**48**:108-118

[38] Liu T, Wang C, Gu X, Gong H, Cheng L, Shi X, et al. Drug delivery with PEGylated MoS2 Nano-sheets for combined photothermal and chemotherapy of cancer. Advanced Materials. 2014;**26**(21):3433-3440

[39] Zhang L, Xia J, Zhao Q, Liu L, Zhang Z. Functional graphene oxide as a nanocarrier for controlled loading and targeted delivery of mixed anticancer drugs. Small. 2010;**6**(4):537-544

[40] Krishna R, Mayer LD. Multidrug resistance (MDR) in cancer: Mechanisms, reversal using modulators of MDR and the role of MDR modulators in influencing the pharmacokinetics of anticancer drugs. European Journal of Pharmaceutical Sciences. 2000;**11**(4):265-283

[41] Brigger I, Dubernet C, Couvreur P. Nanoparticles in cancer therapy and diagnosis. Advanced Drug Delivery Reviews. 2012;**64**:24-36

[42] Astier A, Doat B, Ferrer MJ, Benoit G, Fleury J, Rolland A, et al. Enhancement of adriamycin antitumor activity by its binding with an intracellular sustained-release form, polymethacrylatenanospheres, in U-937 cells. Cancer Research. 1988;**48**(7):1835-1841

[43] Gobin AM, Lee MH, Halas NJ, James WD, Drezek RA, West JL. Near-infrared resonant nanoshells for combined optical imaging and photothermal cancer therapy. Nano Letters. 2007;**7**(7):1929-1934

[44] Yang H, Mao H, Wan Z, Zhu A, Guo M, Li Y, et al. Micelles assembled with carbocyanine dyes for theranostic near-infrared fluorescent cancer imaging and photothermal therapy. Biomaterials. 2013;**34**(36):9124-9133

[45] Yang K, Xu H, Cheng L, Sun C, Wang J, Liu Z. In vitro and in vivo near-infrared photothermal therapy of cancer using polypyrrole organic nanoparticles. Advanced Materials. 2012;**24**(41):5586-5592

[46] Wang YW, Fu YY, Peng Q, Guo SS, Liu G, Li J, et al. Dye-enhanced graphene oxide for photothermal therapy and photoacoustic imaging. Journal of Materials Chemistry B. 2013;**1**(42):5762-5767

[47] Tang J, Jiang X, Wang L, Zhang H, Hu Z, Liu Y, et al. Au@ Pt nanostructures: A novel photothermal conversion agent for cancer therapy. Nanoscale. 2014;**6**(7):3670-3678

[48] Lin Z, Liu Y, Ma X, Hu S, Zhang J, Wu Q, et al. Photothermal ablation of bone metastasis of breast cancer using PEGylated multi-walled carbon nanotubes. Scientific Reports. 2015 Jun 30;**5**:11709

[49] Tu X, Ma Y, Cao Y, Huang J, Zhang M, Zhang Z. PEGylated carbon nanoparticles for efficient in vitro photothermal cancer therapy. Journal of Materials Chemistry B. 2014;**2**(15):2184-2192

[50] Yang K, Zhang S, Zhang G, Sun X, Lee ST, Liu Z. Graphene in mice: Ultrahigh in vivo tumor uptake and efficient photothermal therapy. Nano Letters. 2010;**10**(9):3318-3323

[51] Gupta AK, Gupta M. Cytotoxicity suppression and cellular uptake enhancement of surface modified magnetic nanoparticles. Biomaterials. 2005;**26**(13):1565-1573

[52] Mashal A, Sitharaman B, Li X, Avti PK, Sahakian AV, Booske JH, et al. Toward carbon-nanotube-based theranostic agents for microwave detection and treatment of breast cancer: Enhanced dielectric and heating response of tissue-mimicking materials. IEEE Transactions on Biomedical Engineering. 2010;**57**(8):1831-1834

[53] Huang Z, Xu H, Meyers AD, Musani AI, Wang L, Tagg R, et al. Photodynamic therapy for treatment of solid tumors—Potential and technical challenges. Technology in Cancer Research & Treatment. 2008;**7**(4):309-320

[54] Huang P, Lin J, Wang X, Wang Z, Zhang C, He M, et al. Light-triggered theranostics based on photosensitizer-conjugated carbon dots for simultaneous enhanced-fluorescence imaging and photodynamic therapy. Advanced Materials. 2012;**24**(37):5104-5110

[55] Lucky SS, Soo KC, Zhang Y. Nanoparticles in photodynamic therapy. Chemical Reviews. 2015;**115**(4):1990-2042

[56] Taratula O, Schumann C, Naleway MA, Pang AJ, Chon KJ, Taratula O. A multifunctional theranostic platform based on phthalocyanine-loaded dendrimer for image-guided drug delivery and photodynamic therapy. Molecular Pharmaceutics. 2013;**10**(10):3946-3958

[57] Li Z, Wang C, Cheng L, Gong H, Yin S, Gong Q, et al. PEG-functionalized iron oxide nanoclusters loaded with chlorin e6 for targeted, NIR light induced, photodynamic therapy. Biomaterials. 2013;**34**(36):9160-9170

[58] Park YI, Kim HM, Kim JH, Moon KC, Yoo B, Lee KT, et al. Theranostic probe based on lanthanide-doped nanoparticles for simultaneous in vivo dual-modal imaging and photodynamic therapy. Advanced Materials. 2012;**24**(42):5755-5761

[59] Hainfeld JF, Dilmanian FA, Slatkin DN, Smilowitz HM. Radiotherapy enhancement with gold nanoparticles. Journal of Pharmacy and Pharmacology. 2008;**60**(8):977-985

[60] Rosenberg SA, Restifo NP. Adoptive cell transfer as personalized immunotherapy for human cancer. Science. 2015;**348**(6230):62-68

[61] Mitsunaga M, Nakajima T, Sano K, Choyke PL, Kobayashi H. Near-infrared theranosticphotoimmunotherapy (PIT): Repeated exposure of light enhances the effect of immunoconjugate. Bioconjugate Chemistry. 2012;**23**(3):604-609

[62] Zhang W, Wang Y, Sun X, Wang W, Chen L. Mesoporoustitania based yolk–shell nanoparticles as multifunctional theranostic platforms for SERS imaging and chemo-photothermal treatment. Nanoscale. 2014;**6**(23):14514-14522

[63] Liu J, Wang C, Wang X, Wang X, Cheng L, Li Y, et al. Mesoporous silica coated single-walled carbon nanotubes as a multifunctional light-responsive platform for cancer combination

therapy. Advanced Functional Materials. 2015;**25**(3):384-392

[64] Sahu A, Choi WI, Lee JH, Tae G. Graphene oxide mediated delivery of methylene blue for combined photodynamic and photothermal therapy. Biomaterials. 2013;**34**(26):6239-6248

[65] Gong H, Dong Z, Liu Y, Yin S, Cheng L, Xi W, et al. Engineering of multifunctional nano-micelles for combined photothermal and photodynamic therapy under the guidance of multimodal imaging. Advanced Functional Materials. 2014;**24**(41):6492-6502

[66] Taratula O, Schumann C, Duong T, Taylor KL, Taratula O. Dendrimer-encapsulated naphthalocyanine as a single agent-based theranosticnanoplatform for near-infrared fluorescence imaging and combinatorial anticancer phototherapy. Nanoscale. 2015;7(9):3888-3902

[67] Park H, Yang J, Lee J, Haam S, Choi IH, Yoo KH. Multifunctional nanoparticles for combined doxorubicin and photothermal treatments. ACS Nano. 2009;**3**(10):2919-2926

[68] Jo SD, Ku SH, Won YY, Kim SH, Kwon IC. Targeted nanotheranostics for future personalized medicine: Recent progress in cancer therapy. Theranostics. 2016;**6**(9):1362

[69] Koukourakis Sofia Koukouraki, Alexandra Giatromanolaki, SteliosKakolyris, VassilisGeorgoulias, AntigoniVelidaki, SpyridonArchimandritis and Nikolaos N. Karkavitsas, M.I., 2000. High intratumoral accumulation of stealth liposomal doxorubicin in sarcomas: rationale for combination with radiotherapy. Actaoncologica, 39(2), pp.207-211.

[70] Kircher MF, De La Zerda A, Jokerst JV, Zavaleta CL, Kempen PJ, Mittra E, et al. A brain tumor molecular imaging strategy using a new triple-modality MRI-photoacoustic-Raman nanoparticle. Nature Medicine. 2012;**18**(5):829